"Most of us have heard the expression 'you are what you eat.' Pam Braun has taken this to a new level with her cookbook, *The Ultimate Anti-Cancer Cookbook*. Incorporating sound science, a chef's sensibility, an editor's precision, and common sense, this is a book you will use over and over again—all the while feeling good from enjoying her delicious recipes while knowing you're doing something virtuous for your body. Plus, you'll learn a great deal about nutrition along the way. Enjoy it—I have."

—**John Swartzberg, M.D., FACP**
Clinical Professor, Emeritus, UC Berkeley School of Public Health,
Chair, Editorial Board, UC Berkeley Wellness Center

"*The Ultimate Anti-Cancer Cookbook* contains an incredible number of recipes utilizing fresh and nutritious plant-based foods to create interesting and delicious vegetarian dishes. This cookbook is a must for anyone who wants to eat a diet that contributes to better health and aids in the prevention of chronic illnesses like heart disease and diabetes.

Pam is a cancer survivor who was treated by me and has been cancer-free for many years. She firmly believes that her survival has largely been due to healthy eating practices. Recent guidelines issued by the American Cancer Society in *CA: A Cancer Journal for Clinicians* summarize results from many studies that suggest that adherence to a diet high in plant-based foods and lower in high fat foods may also help reduce the risk of recurrence and increase survival for some cancers. There will be 1.5 million new cancer cases diagnosed this year. The majority of these cancers will be cured. It would be sad, if after fighting and winning the battle with cancer, one ignores the chance to prevent chronic illnesses and possibly recurrence of cancer, because they did not adhere to a program of good nutrition and exercise. Therefore, we highly recommend the use of *The Ultimate Anti-Cancer Cookbook* for helping to achieve better health."

—**Raul R. Mena, M.D.**
Associate Clinical Professor of Medicine at UCLA School of Medicine
Medical Director of the Roy and Patricia Disney Family Cancer Center,
Providence Saint Joseph Medical Center

"The evidence to support a diet rich in vegetables and fruits, low in fats and animal proteins is steadily evolving. Pam's careful discussion of the benefits of certain foods and the potential harm of others is thoughtful and balanced. In addition, she has investigated food preparation data as it relates to cancer and included this often overlooked topic in her cookbook. As a cancer doctor for women, I found this cookbook to be a wealth of delicious and healthy recipes that I will be recommending!"

—**BJ Rimel M.D.**
Associate Director for Gynecologic Oncology Clinical Trials, Division of Gynecologic Oncology
Women's Cancer Program, Cedars-Sinai Medical Center

"Pam Braun has written an excellent and informed cookbook that is full of delicious and healthy recipes. As a survivor she brings a personal approach to how selecting colorful fruits and vegetables and a plant based diet may reduce the risk of cancer. I found the Appendices especially helpful as they identify the science behind the food choices she makes. I highly recommend this new addition to the cancer cookbook shelf."

—**Carolyn Katzin, M.S., CNS**
Integrative Oncology Specialist Simms/Mann–UCLA Center for Integrative Oncology

"I loudly applaud *The Ultimate Anti-Cancer Cookbook*, written by a cancer survivor to educate and entertain the consumer. I have known Pam since her cancer diagnosis. During her chemotherapy treatments, and after she was cancer-free, she would often inquire about what type of diet she should incorporate into her lifestyle. Like so many people living with and surviving cancer, the ability to enhance recovery and potentially prevent a cancer recurrence with food and lifestyle choices becomes very empowering. However, the information on the benefits or harm of specific foods and additives is data challenged. Pam's cookbook provides evidence based information to help the consumer make informed decisions. It is user friendly with flavorful, appealing, multi-ethnic food and recipe selections. I am proud to recommend this well done cookbook for healthy living."

—**Paula J. Anastasia RN, MN, AOCN**
Gyn-Oncology Clinical Nurse Specialist, Cedars-Sinai Medical Center

"It is not often that one can remark on such a well-written book as this. While it is true that you are what you eat, that is never more so than in this case. Patients with ovarian cancer need more than one medical miracle and certainly this just adds to the recipe of miracles. It is a pleasure to read this book. It is even more so to actually cook the food as written in this book. Very few of us can say that our life has been enhanced by something such as this, but I can honestly say this is true in this case. As an associate professor in gynecological oncology, it is unusual to encounter someone with both the intellect and the artistic endeavor, as demonstrated in this book of recipes. I highly recommend both from the hunger point of view and the artistic point of view as well."

—**Ronald S. Leuchter, M.D.**
Clinical Associate Professor, Obstetrics and Gynecology, and Gynecologic Oncology
David Geffen School of Medicine, UCLA, Los Angeles, CA

"Pam Braun's cookbook is a great resource from one survivor to another. These straightforward healthy recipes will help either a newly diagnosed patient or a longer term survivor take control of their diet and make healthy choices at a critical time."

— **Mary L. Hardy, M.D.**
Former medical director of the Simms/Mann UCLA Center for Integrative Oncology
Board Member of the Society of Integrative Oncology

"I witnessed the early, middle, and late stages of Pam's life-threatening battle with fallopian tube cancer. To my grateful astonishment, my friend survived with an energy, vitality, and enthusiasm unique to our twelve-year social and professional relationship. With all respect to modern medicine, Pam credits extensive dietary research leading to these new and innovative ideas for food preparation. Perhaps Pam has inadvertently given birth to a whimsical new adage, 'If it's broke, fix it.'"

—**Dabney Coleman**

"Read it. Eat it. You'll love it!"   —**Tuesday Weld**

"If you are on your own cancer journey, I hope this book will help you through it. If you are not on a cancer journey, I hope this book will deter you from taking the trip in the first place."

Estimated Percentage Of Cancers and Number of Cases That Could Be Prevented in the U.S. Yearly by Eating a Healthy Diet, Getting Regular Physical Activity, and Maintaining a Healthy Weight

50% of colon cancers (72,000 cases)
38% of female breast cancers (86,000 cases)
70% of endometrial cancers (33,000 cases)
69% of esophogeal cancers (12,000 cases)
21% of gall bladder cancers (2,000 cases)
15% of liver cancers (4,000 cases)
24% of kidney cancers (16,000 cases)
36% of lung cancers that are not caused by tobacco (3,600-7,200 cases)
63% of mouth, pharynx and larynx cancers (33,000 cases)
19% of pancreatic cancers (8,300 cases)
47% of stomach cancers (10,000 cases)
11% of prostate cancers (26,250 cases)

Estimates based upon the findings of the 2007 American Institute for Cancer Research and World Cancer Research Fund's Second Expert Report and updates.

The Ultimate Anti-Cancer Cookbook

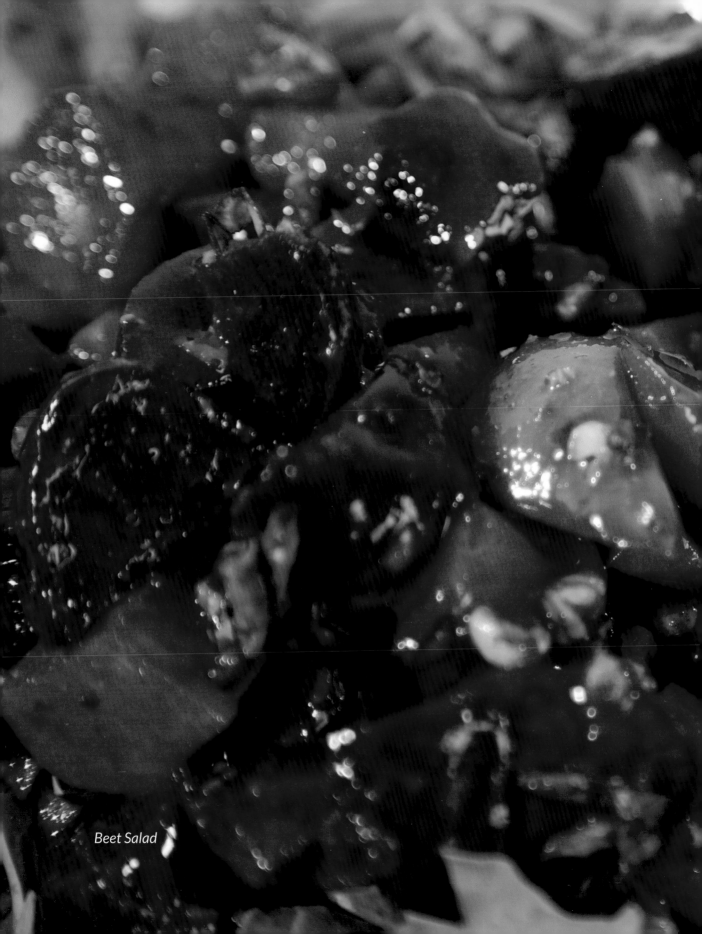

Beet Salad

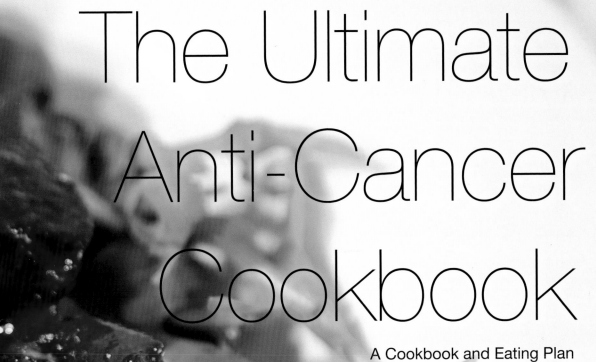

The Ultimate Anti-Cancer Cookbook

A Cookbook and Eating Plan
Developed by a Late-Stage
Cancer Survivor with
225 Delicious Recipes
for Everyday Meals,
Using Everyday Foods

PAM BRAUN
Photographs by Robert Sobul

THIS IS A GENUINE VIREO BOOK

V

A Vireo Book | Rare Bird Books
453 South Spring Street, Suite 531
Los Angeles, CA 90013
rarebirdbooks.com

If you are already fighting cancer, this book does not constitute medical advice. If you have cancer, it should be used as a supplement to conventional cancer treatments or alternative cancer treatments, not as a substitute for them.

Whether you are fighting cancer or not, please consult with your physician before making any dietary changes. Following the advice in this book does not constitute a guarantee of a disease-free life.

Photographs by Robert Sobul
Author photograph by Liz Sterling

Set in Lato
Printed in Canada
Distributed in the U.S. by Publishers Group West

10 9 8 7 6 5 4 3 2 1

Publisher's Cataloging-in-Publication data

Braun, Pam, 1952 —

    The Ultimate anti-cancer cookbook : a cookbook and eating plan developed by a late-stage cancer survivor with 225 delicious recipes for everyday meals , using everyday foods / by Pam Braun
    p. cm.
    ISBN 978-0988745612
    Includes bibliographical references.

1. Cancer—Diet therapy—Recipes. 2. Cancer—Nutritional aspects. 3. Cancer—Prevention. I. The Ultimate anti-cancer cookbook : a cookbook and eating plan developed by a late-stage cancer survivor with two hundred and twenty five delicious recipes for everyday meals , using everyday foods. II. Title.

RC271.D52 B72 2013
616.99/40654 -dc23

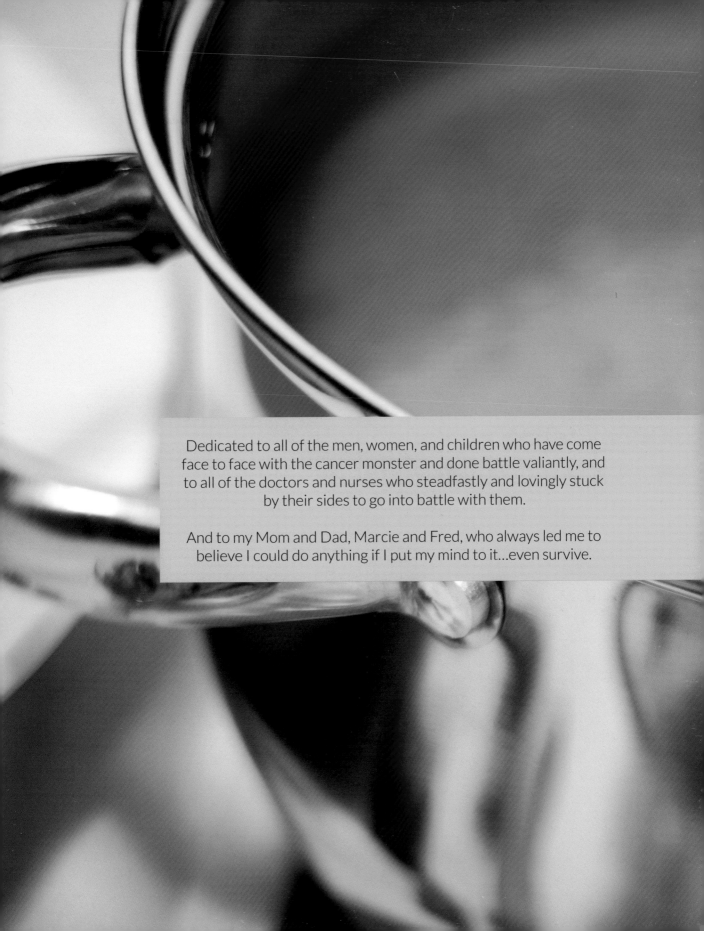

Dedicated to all of the men, women, and children who have come face to face with the cancer monster and done battle valiantly, and to all of the doctors and nurses who steadfastly and lovingly stuck by their sides to go into battle with them.

And to my Mom and Dad, Marcie and Fred, who always led me to believe I could do anything if I put my mind to it...even survive.

"In the summer of 2004, at the age of 52, I was not feeling well. The fact is that I was almost dead and didn't know it."

Garlic Bread

Contents

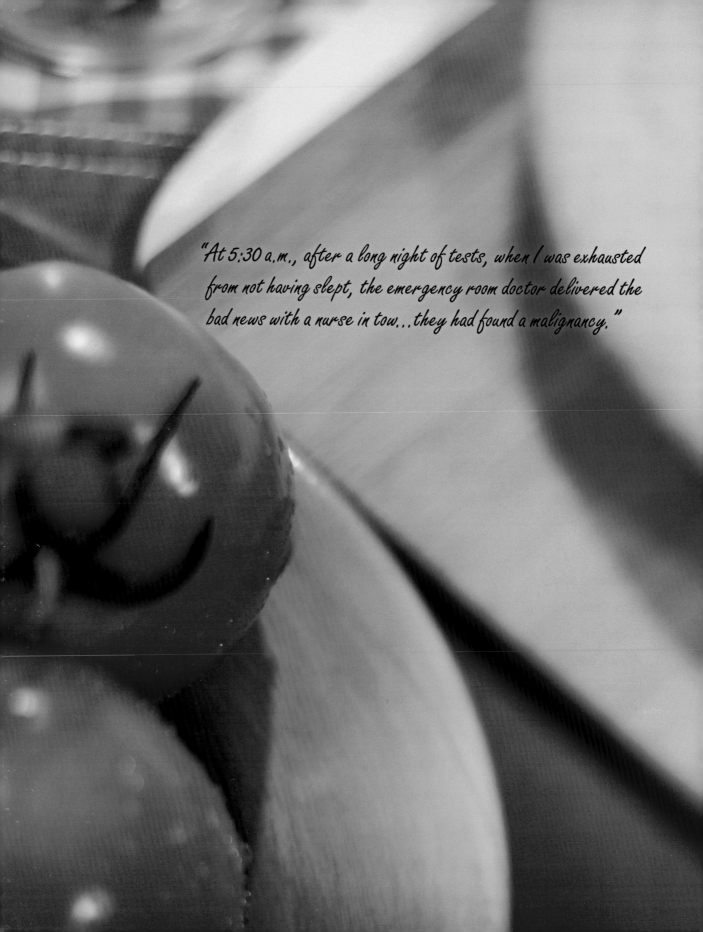

"At 5:30 a.m., after a long night of tests, when I was exhausted from not having slept, the emergency room doctor delivered the bad news with a nurse in tow...they had found a malignancy."

Foreword

By Jodi Newson, MS, RD, CSO, Director of Nutrition Services
Tower Hematology/Oncology Medical Group, Los Angeles, CA
Master of Science in Nutritional Science, Registered Dietitian,
Board Certified Specialist in Oncology Nutrition

Cookbooks come in all types. Some focus on regional cuisines, some advocate certain diet plans, and others are built around a single ingredient. However different they all may be, the common denominator is the creation of food (or, in some instances, what passes as food).

This cookbook is really about health. It's about nourishing your body with phytochemicals and nutrients that aid your body in fighting disease. It isn't by someone "famous" who espouses the next new thing. There are no celebrity chefs behind the scenes. There is just Pam—who made a commitment to life when the odds were stacked against her.

As a Board Certified Specialist in Oncology Nutrition, I spend a lot of time disseminating myth from fact. Science is constantly evolving, and so too are opinions of what foods are beneficial. There is definitely gray area out there, but there are also numerous scientific studies supporting the disease-fighting powers of certain foods.

According to the National Cancer Institute, one in two people born today will be diagnosed with cancer (based on cancer rates from 2005-2007). If we know that eating a largely plant-based diet can aid in the prevention of cancer, heart disease, diabetes, and other chronic illnesses (and we *do* know this via scientific research), why wouldn't we *all* try to eat this way? What do we have to lose? We may lose weight, and we may also gain greater health and longevity.

There are no guarantees that eating well and exercising will provide you with a disease-free existence. However, when we know that eating poorly and being sedentary may lead to disease, the choice seems obvious. Eat well!

You will find so many delicious, hearty, and healthful recipes in this cookbook that will satisfy everyone. There truly is something for everyone—even the die-hard meat-and-potatoes types will be impressed.

So ask yourself this, "Why wouldn't I do everything in my power to be healthy and prevent disease?" You have the power to help prevent cancer and other chronic illnesses. As a healthcare practitioner, I highly recommend that you use it.

"My doctor gave me a 15% chance of survival. I sat at my dining room table, shell-shocked and numb. Then I thought, 'Wait a minute. When have I not come into the top 15% of anything once I put my mind to it?'"

Introduction

I recently went to a reunion and during the in memoriam section, as the pictures of those no longer with us flashed up on the screen, a friend leaned over to me and whispered in my ear, "Just think, your picture could be up there." He didn't need to remind me. I was already thinking of that and counting my blessings. I am a late-stage cancer survivor who defied the odds and in all probability shouldn't still be here. But I am, and I believe with all of my heart that food is a major reason I survived to write this book.

In the summer of 2004, I was diagnosed with late-stage cancer and given the estimate of a 15% chance of survival by my doctor. I knew there wasn't much about the cancer journey that I could control, but I was going to make the most out of what I could control, mainly diet and exercise. I immediately started a continuing research project on foods and their relationships to cancer, and found this to be true: *Some foods have been scientifically shown to help prevent certain cancers, and other foods have been scientifically shown to help cause certain cancers.* Studies have confirmed that specific nutrition does help prevent certain cancers, but not shown it for other cancers...yet. The evidence to date is inconclusive for some cancers, but that doesn't mean it might not prove positive at some date in the future. In the meantime, it is reasonable to follow as healthy a diet as we can.

If you've picked up this book, you probably have cancer or know someone who does. Quite frankly, who doesn't? According to the American Cancer Society, "Cancer is the general name for a group of more than 100 diseases in which cells in a part of the body begin to grow out of control." Although we tend to take it in stride as we live our lives, in fact it's an epidemic. Like an elephant in the middle of the room, we ignore it and walk around it until we are forced to deal with it. We think that maybe if we ignore it, it will go away. Cancer is still the dreaded "C" word. Everyone's afraid to say it, to talk about it. Unfortunately, it's not going anywhere. The elephant is only getting bigger. I hear it all of the time: "My mother, my sister, my father-in-law, my son, my dog..." No one is immune to this monster. It will eventually touch all of us in one way or another. And yet, we keep tiptoeing around it hoping it won't happen to us, but it can. When the dreaded diagnosis is heard, most people will do anything to help themselves. Why not start before you have to go through what I did? Before your children have to go through what I did?

Studies now show that if you are female and reading this book, you have a one in three chance of getting cancer in your lifetime. Not your neighbor or your co-worker—you. Don't think it's always going to be somebody else. The fact is, you have a good chance of getting it. If you're male or a newborn, it's even worse. You have a one in two chance of getting it. Children being born today are up against terrible 50/50 odds of getting cancer in their lifetimes unless changes are made.

There is some light amongst the darkness here. According to the report in the online journal *Cancer* (March, 2012), the U.S. Centers for Disease Control and Prevention, the American Cancer Society, the National Cancer Institute, and the North American Association of Central Cancer Registries, death rates for all cancers including the four most common (lung, colorectal, breast, and prostate) have steadily declined from 1999 to 2008. The decline in both deaths and new cases of cancer is believed to be from better scientific understanding of how to diagnose, treat, and prevent cancer in the first place.

Which means we aren't helpless against it—far from it. Especially if we start now, before the dreaded diagnosis, while we are still healthy. The reality is that cancer is no longer considered the luck of the draw, or due primarily to genetics. In actuality, only a very small amount of all cancers are due to inherited predispositions from our ancestors. Many cancers are caused by environment, diet, and lack of exercise. A study conducted by the University of Copenhagen and described in the *New England Journal of Medicine* in March of 1988 reported that children who were adopted at birth had early mortality rates (including cancer) consistent with their adoptive parents. There was no association between early mortality rates and birth parents.

You might be thinking, *Who are you to tell me how to prevent cancer? You got it!* That's correct, I did, but I didn't get it back again when the odds were heavily stacked against me—and I believe it was my diet and exercise program that have prevented a recurrence. At this time, scientific data is inconclusive as to whether diet can significantly help prevent a cancer recurrence. Still, the American Cancer Society recently released recommended guidelines to promote a healthy lifestyle for cancer survivors. They have long promoted these recommendations to help prevent certain cancers, but they now suggest the same guidelines for cancer survivors to help prevent cancer recurrence.

Their recommendations are to stay away from tobacco, maintain a healthy weight, exercise, limit time spent sitting—and eat fruits, vegetables, and whole grains. They also recommend limiting your intake of red meat, processed meat, and alcohol. These are the same points that I recommend in my eating plan.

There is strong evidence that a plant-based diet cuts the risk of cancer overall, so I personally chose to err on the side of caution, and now the American Cancer Society concurs. I chose to create and eat a diet centered around foods that have been shown to help prevent cancer, even though scientific studies were and are still underway regarding their effectiveness in recurrence avoidance.

The fact is we don't know for sure why some folks will get cancer and others won't, or why some cancer survivors have a recurrence and others don't. But we're learning more all of the time. In the meantime, it continues to make sense that keeping your body as healthy as possible at all times—including before, during, and after the cancer process—helps to fight off the disease. Although scientific proof is still emerging, I believe that it is better for your body and more cancer-preventative to eat a fresh salad than a glazed donut.

Years ago, I had my head in the sand thinking that cancer is the kind of thing that happens to other people, not me. I was middle-aged and slightly overweight. I didn't eat that poorly, but my diet wasn't that terrific, either. I hardly exercised and had a lot of stress in my life. I always heard the latest news about which food was bad for me or which food was good for me, but quite frankly it went in one ear and out the other. "Blah, blah, blah, what will they tell me is bad for me next?" I blithely went through life eating whatever I wanted, buying larger sized clothing as middle age crept in, always assuming the Big C was not going to come knocking on my door. Looking back on it now, it was just a matter of time for me.

My original (incorrect) preliminary cancer diagnosis was lymphoma; the cancer was in so many lymph nodes it presented itself as lymphoma. Later, after more tests, I was diagnosed with late-stage fallopian tube cancer. It was estimated by my doctor that I had a 15% chance of survival. Six months later, after conventional treatment, I managed to get clean from the disease (as many women do). I was then given the estimate of a 75% chance of a recurrence by my doctor. That's what makes late-stage ovarian/fallopian tube cancer so lethal. Sure, you can get clean from it, but staying clean is the near impossible part. It is not unusual for women to *get* cancer-free from this disease. It is unusual to *stay* cancer-free from this disease.

Because of the high recurrence rate within the first three years for ovarian/fallopian tube cancer, drug companies are working on drugs that would halt the recurrences. I was involved in a clinical trial that was conducted in hospitals around the country for one of these hopeful drugs. After nine months, the study was shut down because it was clear the drug was not working—too many women in the study had relapsed. I was the only woman in the trial at my hospital who had not.

One online friend involved in the same clinical trial once said to me, "Oh, I could never give up meat. I'd die if I had to give up meat." What she should have said is, "I'll die if I don't give up meat." But she didn't, and she did. I know that I was given a second chance at life. After literally years of food research and walking the walk, I have been and remain cancer-free. I have never had a recurrence.

There is plenty of scientific evidence out there showing that eating right can help prevent cancer, and eating incorrectly can help cause cancer. Although scientific evidence is still mixed, and studies are still underway regarding foods preventing a recurrence, I believe that diet and lifestyle are keeping me cancer-free. The odds were stacked against me, yet here I am, feeling as good or better than I did in my twenties. Scientific evidence has established that diet and exercise can significantly reduce the odds of getting cancer in the first place.

Eating, of course, needs to be a pleasurable activity to the senses, as well as a healthy one for the body. I purposely wanted to create a cookbook full of delicious recipes that would appeal to people who liked to eat good food—not a "health food" book. I created a cookbook that uses everyday foods for everyday families because not everyone has the time or the money to visit the health food stores or the farmer's markets, but everyone might get cancer.

I've always loved to eat, and I've always loved to cook too! I am a bit of a pro—I have a long history of being in the restaurant business owning, managing, and cooking. Quite frankly, food and I are old friends. Now, I have arranged my kitchen and my life around cancer prevention. With a little bit of effort, you can too.

A Note About Studies

Cancer-Fighting Foods: Please note that when I reference a food that has been found to help fight cancer, the information may have come from several sources. The results may have come from laboratory tests using animals, laboratory tests using human cells, clinical trials involving humans who might have had their eating habits monitored, or from interviews with people about their personal eating habits.

Keep in mind, also, that a food may have been found to help prevent or fight a specific type of cancer, but not necessarily all cancers. Please see *Appendix-I* for some studies that have been cited, and *Appendix-II* for the American Cancer Society's Guideline on Nutrition for Cancer Prevention and Cancer Survivors. The Guideline includes the Society's basic recommendations on nutrition to help fight or prevent all cancers, along with specific recommendations for specific cancers.

Additionally, please see *Appendix-III* for the results of the Second Expert Report published by the World Health Research Fund and the American Institute for Cancer Research, *Food, Nutrition, Physical Activity, and the Prevention of Cancer: A Global Perspective.* These results indicate which foods have been shown through studies to either decrease or increase the risk of specific cancers in varying degrees.

How To Use This Book

Congratulations on obtaining and reading this book! It means you are ready to make a change in your diet to avoid getting cancer. Change is hard, I get that. I also get that dealing with cancer and chemotherapy and/or radiation is hard, so change is the better of the two choices.

The changes that I'm suggesting might be difficult to undertake all at once. Start slowly, start somewhere, but start! Your life probably depends on it. We are in a middle of a cancer epidemic. Cancer kills 1,500 Americans a day, and has unfortunately become an accepted American way of life, but it doesn't have to be. It is estimated that one-third of American cancer deaths could be prevented by diet and exercise. At one time we stood by helplessly as we thought, *It's out of my control* or *It's in my genes*. New studies have begun to show that cancer is not the luck of the draw, or purely genetic, as we previously thought. In actuality, less than 10% of cancers are hereditary or genetic.

The way to use this book is very simple:

- Try to include the foods in the Foods to Enjoy chapter in what you eat every day.
- Avoid the foods in the Foods to Avoid chapter.
- Use the Preparation Tips to prepare your foods correctly for optimal health benefits.

Pretty simple and a whole lot easier than dealing with cancer!

The more you eat properly, the easier it will become. At one time, I loved a double cheeseburger and a shake. Now, I couldn't eat it if it were sitting in front of me. My body changed, and my tastes changed. I no longer crave the unhealthy foods, and I now crave the healthy foods, but it didn't happen overnight. It took me a while to get to the place where the thought of a double cheeseburger no longer makes me salivate, but I did get here. Over the last few years (as I've tweaked my diet) if I ever got a really bad craving for something, I'd enjoy it and get it out of my system. Now, that rarely happens to me. I crave what's good for me, not what's bad for me, and you can get here, too.

You don't have to dive right in and change your eating habits 180 degrees immediately. That's too drastic, and you probably won't stick to it unless you have cancer—then you'll do anything. I know, I've been there. My diet is continually changing as I continue to read and research. I started out by not eating red meat. Then I gave up any and all junk food. Then I gave up even chicken and fish, while only occasionally indulging in a piece of salmon or chicken breast. The change has been steady and slow. Now I eat a 98% vegan diet. This was my choice, this is where I ended up, but it would have been way too drastic to do in one fell swoop. Start by making subtle changes to get started, especially if you're a meat and potatoes kind of person.

- Switch to a vegetarian meal one night a week (make it interesting, not boring).
- Start reducing your red meat intake and replace it with chicken or fish.
- While weaning your diet off meat, start cooking meats and fish over a low heat, not a high heat, and avoid searing, charring or placing meat and fish over a direct flame.
- Eat a salad for lunch one day a week instead of a lunch-meat sandwich. Try to wean yourself off of lunch-meat altogether.
- Ditch the iceberg lettuce when making salads or sandwiches and replace it with hearty greens such as spinach, kale, arugula, or collard greens.
- Start using olive oil and balsamic vinegar on your salads instead of fat and sugar-laden, store-bought salad dressings.
- Give up the cookies or chips for a snack one day a week and switch to a handful of almonds and raisins. The goal is to eventually stop eating junk food altogether.
- Try a piece of dark chocolate for dessert instead of cake or pie.
- If you're a soda drinker, start weaning yourself off of sodas.
- Avoid deep-fried foods.
- Switch the sugar-filled cereal in the morning to a healthy sugar-free and artificial-sweetener-free cereal with fresh berries.
- Start taking a ten minute walk before dinner every night, and gradually increase the time.

The more you do it, the easier it will become. Most of us are creatures of habit, and it's a matter of changing our old routines and our old habits to newer, healthier ones.

Stop thinking of your meal plate as consisting of meat, potato, and vegetables, and start thinking outside of your food comfort zone. The USDA has a new food pyramid made up of more whole grains, fruits and vegetables, less meat, and more beans. The new food plate recommended by the American Institute for Cancer Research consists of two-thirds vegetables and one-third (or less) meat or fish.

Also, know and accept that there will be more time spent in the kitchen. Eating properly does take some prep work, but it's worth it. Getting and dealing with cancer ate up six months of my life. Talk about time consumption! A little extra time in the kitchen cleaning or prepping some vegetables? No problem in comparison.

I love to cook and I love to eat, so the recipes in this book are varied and all over the map. My personal daily menu is somewhat limited for breakfasts and lunches, since that is the way I choose to get my Foods to Enjoy in, and my variety usually comes with dinner. You can mix and match these recipes however you like to get the end result. Just try to include the Foods to Enjoy every day, prepared properly, and avoid the Foods to Avoid.

Acknowledgments

Thanks to all who supported me and encouraged me throughout this endeavor, especially Liz Sterling and Gail Berry, who spent hours researching and slaving over hot computers. A heartfelt thank you goes out to Jodi Newson, Dr. John Swartzberg, and Marianne Moloney for allowing me to pick their brains and for time and attention given. Of course, I want to thank my talented doctors for saving my life so I could write this book at all: Dr. Raul Mena, Dr. Ronald Leuchter, and Dr. Deborah Anderson. Last, but not least, a very special thank you goes out to all of my family and friends who helped all across the country in their "test kitchens": Reverend Sheila Christly, Yvonne Ghareeb, Donna Hart, Marty Stevens-Heebner, Betty Kaplan, Jen Kramer, Patty La Due, John LaMartine, Steve Lundquist, Alexis Lyman, Marianne Moloney, Ellen and Steve Peters, Lynn Roberts, Shar Sandera, Susan Silberberg, Marianne Simpson, Mandy Vento, Kay Walbye.

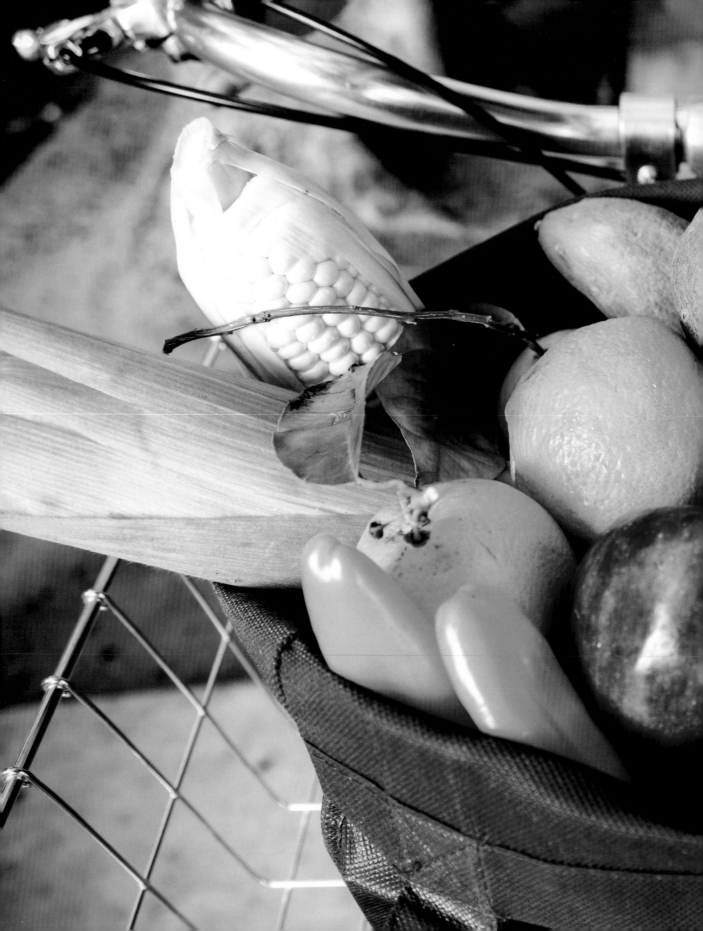

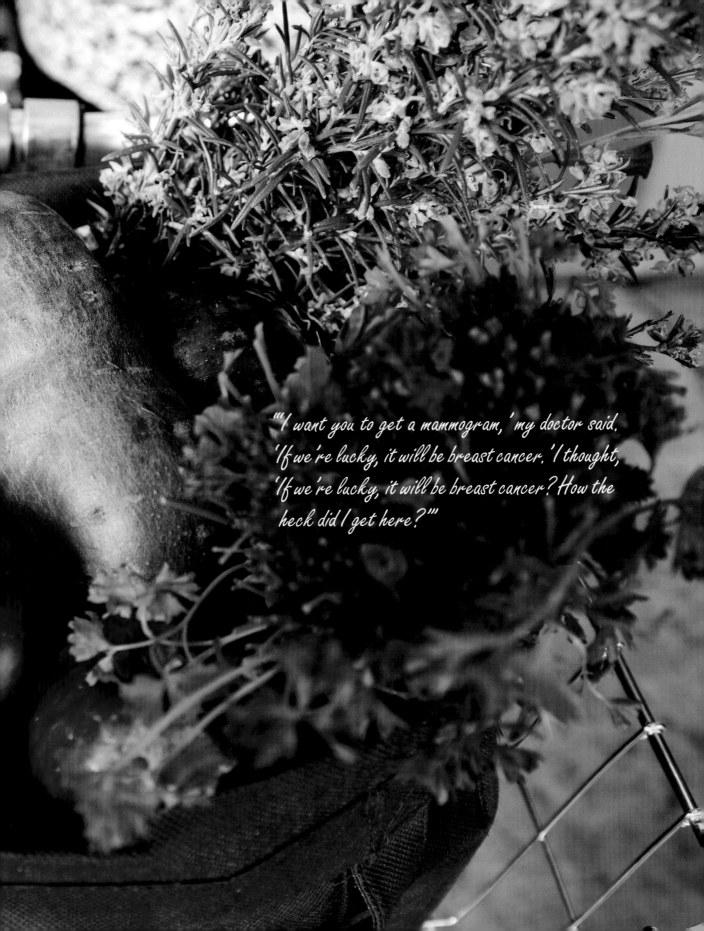

"'I want you to get a mammogram,' my doctor said, 'If we're lucky, it will be breast cancer.' I thought, 'If we're lucky, it will be breast cancer? How the heck did I get here?'"

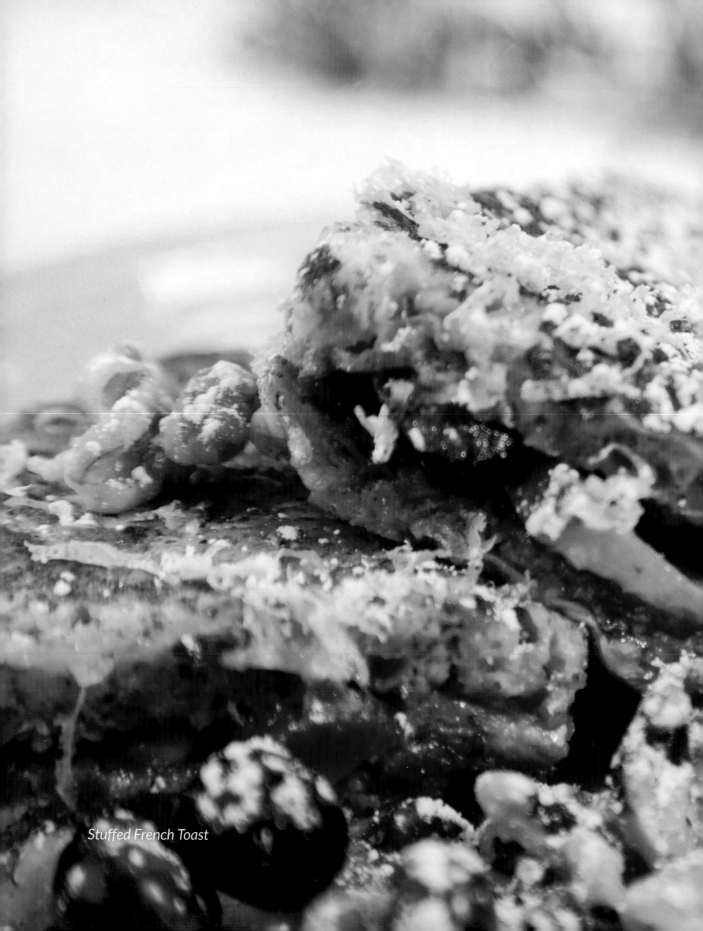

Stuffed French Toast

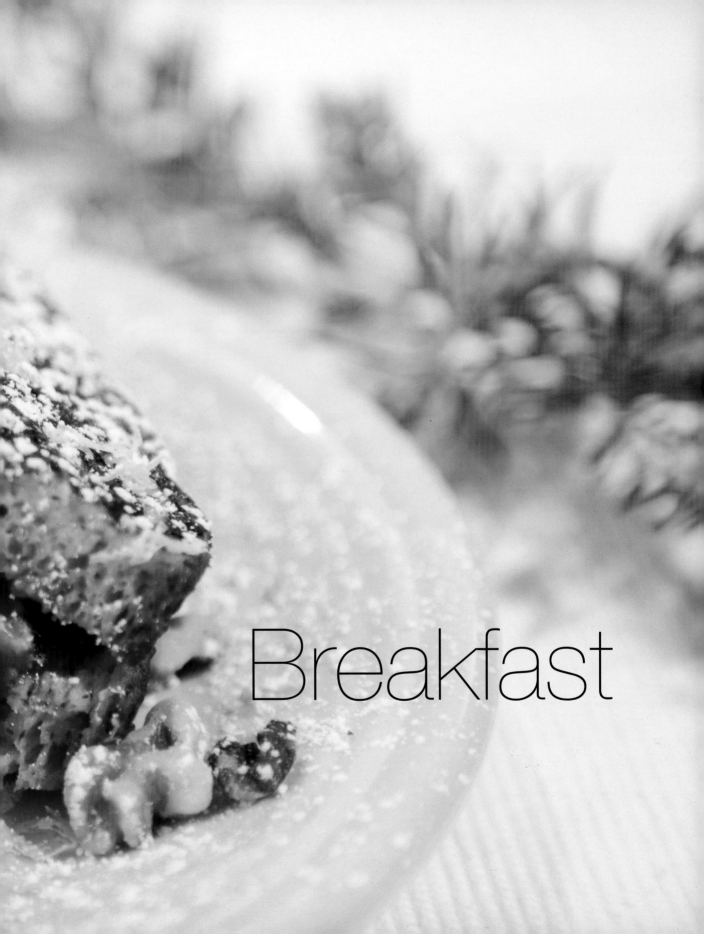

Breakfast

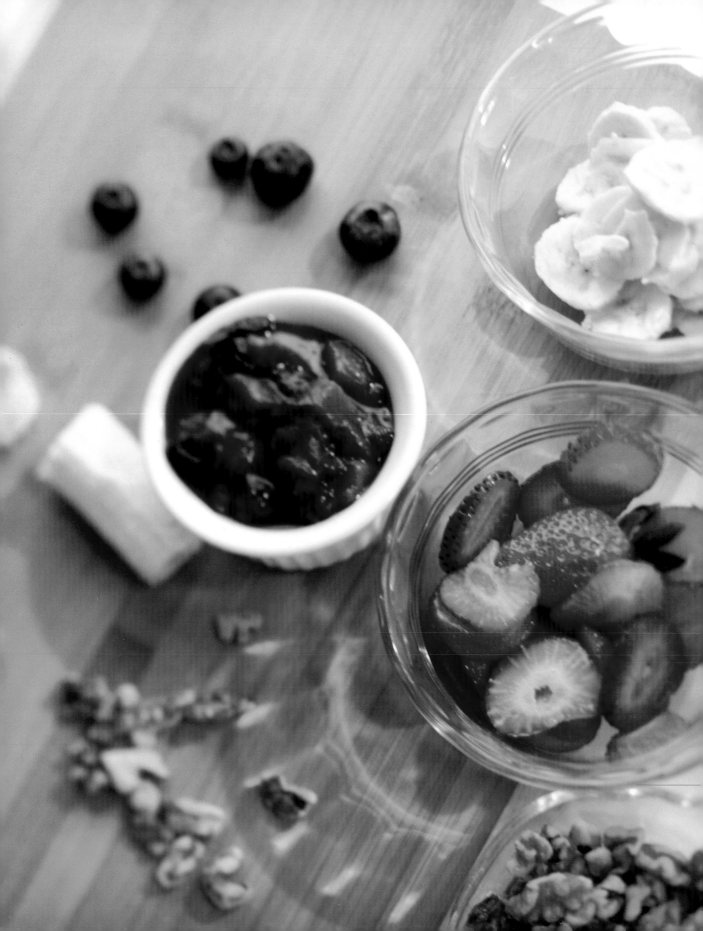

You'll notice this section is relatively small. That's because I, like most people, tend to eat the same thing for breakfast every day. I usually have a bowl of whole grain cereal, topped with some banana, berries, and soy milk. I do this for two reasons: the time constraints involved in getting ready for work on a weekday morning, and because whole grain cereal and fruit are healthier choices. On the weekends when I have more time, I enjoy a little more variety and fun with breakfasts. Again, I do this in moderation only.

The problem with most traditional breakfasts is that they typically contain unhealthy fats, processed meats, and sugars. Never fear, we can still enjoy tasty breakfasts! The recipes in this section are healthier versions of familiar favorites.

Egg Whites Florentine English Muffins

This might satisfy a craving for Eggs Benedict without sacrificing your health. Jam packed with spinach, these open-faced sandwiches are a welcome Sunday morning treat!

2 whole wheat English muffins
¼ cup shredded cheese (part-skim mozzarella, veggie, or soy)
2 tablespoons canola oil
4 cups fresh spinach, loosely packed, chopped
8 egg whites
1 tablespoon chopped pimento

1 tablespoon cornstarch
¾ cup nonfat milk
1 teaspoon lemon juice
1 tablespoon chopped fresh flat-leaf parsley
Salt and pepper
Canola oil spray

Preheat oven to 250 degrees F. Split the muffins and toast lightly. Place pieces side by side on a cookie sheet. Spread cheese evenly over the muffins and put in preheated oven to melt.

In a medium skillet, over medium-high heat, sauté spinach in 1 tablespoon canola oil until spinach wilts. Salt and pepper to taste and set aside.

Spray another medium skillet with canola oil spray and place over a low heat. Add the egg whites. Sprinkle the chopped pimento over the eggs. Cover the skillet until eggs are cooked (to allow the eggs to get fluffly). Remove cover, remove from heat, and set aside.

Place the sautéed spinach on top of the muffins. Put the eggs on top of the spinach. Place cookie sheet back into the oven to keep warm.

In a small skillet, whisk together the cornstarch and 1 tablespoon canola oil until the cornstarch dissolves. Place skillet over a high heat. Whisking constantly, slowly add the milk until the mixture begins to boil and thicken. Reduce heat and continue cooking, still whisking constantly for 1 minute. Remove from heat. Whisk in the lemon juice and parsley. Salt and pepper to taste.

Remove muffins from oven and place on serving plates. Pour white sauce evenly over muffins. Serve with fresh, seasonal fruit on the side.

Note: Whisk in a little more milk if white sauce gets too thick. Sauce will thicken if not served immediately.

Serves 4

Eggs Florentine

Occasionally I get a craving for a whole egg, and this recipe satisfies it. It tastes rich and decadent, and is still relatively low-fat. In the past, I would have eaten 2 eggs for breakfast. Now I'm satisfied with one...and only on occasion.

2 tablespoons canola oil
2 tablespoons finely chopped onion
4 cups fresh spinach, loosely packed, chopped
2 tablespoons shredded cheese (part-skim mozzarella, veggie, or soy)
1 tablespoon cornstarch
¾ cup nonfat milk

1 teaspoon low-fat grated Parmesan cheese
1 tablespoon chopped fresh flat-leaf parsley
Salt and pepper
Canola oil spray
2 eggs
Salt and pepper

Preheat oven to 250 degrees F. Over a medium-high heat, in a medium-sized skillet, sauté onions in 1 tablespoon canola oil. Cook until onions are soft. Add spinach and cook until spinach wilts. Salt and pepper to taste. Spoon spinach mixture equally into 2 oven-safe au gratin dishes (or onto 2 oven-safe plates). Sprinkle 1 tablespoon shredded cheese over each spinach mixture and place in preheated oven.

In a small skillet, whisk together the cornstarch and 1 tablespoon canola oil until the cornstarch dissolves. Place skillet over a high heat. Whisking constantly, slowly add the milk until the mixture begins to boil and thicken. Reduce heat and continue cooking, still whisking constantly for 1 minute. Remove from heat. Whisk in Parmesan cheese and parsley. Salt and pepper to taste. Set aside.

Spray a non-stick skillet with canola oil spray. Place skillet over a very low heat, and break 2 eggs into the skillet, being careful not to break yolks. Cover the skillet and cook until eggs are done, but yolks are still soft. Remove cover from eggs and remove skillet from heat.

Carefully remove spinach from the oven. Place 1 egg on top of spinach on each plate. Pour sauce even over each egg. Serve immediately.

Serves 2

Breakfast Burrito

Quick and easy to prepare, this burrito can even be eaten on the go if you leave off the sauce at the end.

1 medium onion, diced
½ medium green pepper, diced
½ medium red pepper, diced
1 tomato, diced
8 egg whites + 2 whole eggs (whisked)
4 10-inch whole wheat flour tortillas
4 ounces shredded cheese (part-skim mozzarella, veggie, or soy)

Salt and pepper
¼ teaspoon hot chili pepper, diced finely (optional)
Canola oil spray
½ cup salsa
1 avocado, peeled and sliced
½ cup plain nonfat yogurt

Preheat oven to 300 degrees F. Spray a medium skillet very well with canola oil spray. Place onion, peppers, and tomato into the sprayed skillet and sauté until onions are translucent and peppers are soft (about 5 minutes). Add eggs and cook until done. Add hot chili pepper if desired. Salt and pepper to taste. Warm tortillas either in the microwave or on the stove top. Place egg mixture in warm tortilla and add cheese. Roll up to form burrito. Place burritos in the preheated oven for 3 minutes to melt cheese. Remove from oven and top with salsa and avocado. Serve nonfat yogurt on the side.

Serves 4

Veggie Egg White Omelet

Covering the omelet keeps in steam and makes it nice and fluffy. You won't miss the yolk!

1 small onion, chopped finely
½ red pepper, chopped finely
1 cup of mushrooms, sliced
1 medium tomato, chopped finely
½ green pepper, chopped finely
5 egg whites plus 1 egg

2 tablespoons chopped flat-leaf parsley
1 tablespoon low-fat grated Parmesan cheese
Salt and pepper
Canola oil spray
¼ cup salsa (optional)

Spray a medium skillet with canola oil spray and place over medium heat. Add onions, peppers, and mushrooms and cook until soft (about 5 minutes). Add tomato and salt and pepper to taste. Cook another 2 minutes, and remove from heat. In a medium bowl, whisk the egg whites and egg until frothy, and pour into a medium skillet sprayed with canola oil spray. Place the skillet on a very low heat. Cover with a tight lid. When the eggs have begun to cook, but are still soft, add the cooked vegetables and sprinkle the parsley and the Parmesan over the vegetables. Replace the cover and continue cooking until eggs are done. Using a spatula, fold the omelette. Cut in half, serve with salsa if desired.

Serves 2

Breakfast Pizza

This is a fun breakfast, or even a fun supper for that matter!

One rolled out 12-inch *Whole Wheat Pizza Dough*
Cornmeal for dusting
1 tablespoon canola oil
½ medium red onion, chopped
½ cup fresh mushrooms, sliced
2 cups fresh spinach, chopped
1 baked potato, precooked and diced into ½ inch pieces

6 egg whites
2 tablespoons chopped flat-leaf parsley
¾ cup shredded cheese (part-skim mozzarella, veggie, or soy)
Canola oil spray
Salt and pepper
½ cup salsa (optional)
Hot pepper flakes (optional)

Preheat oven to 400 degrees F. Sprinkle a pizza paddle with a little cornmeal. Place the rolled out pizza dough onto the paddle. If you don't own a pizza paddle, place the pizza dough onto a cooling rack that is at least as large as the rolled out dough.

Using the paddle, slide the dough directly onto the oven rack in the center of the oven. If using a cooling rack, place the cooling rack in the center of the oven. Cook until dough is slightly firm, about 3 minutes. This will allow you to easily slide the pizza off of the paddle or cooling rack once the toppings are on it. When the dough is slightly firm, remove from oven. Do not turn oven off.

In a medium skillet, sauté the onion in the canola oil until caramelized (about 20 minutes, onions should be soft and slightly brown). Add the mushrooms, spinach, and potato. Cook until the spinach is wilted and the potatoes have some color. Add the egg whites and continue cooking, stirring until the egg whites are scrambled. Salt and pepper to taste.

Spread the egg mixture over the pizza crust, leaving a 1/2-inch border. Top with the chopped parsley and sprinkle with cheese. Return to oven and cook until the crust is crisp and the cheese melts, about 7-10 minutes. Remove from oven, slice, and enjoy! Top with salsa and/or hot pepper flakes if desired.

Serves 2

Cornmeal Pancakes

I eat cereal with berries and soy milk almost every day for breakfast. On the weekends, I sometimes like to have pancakes as a treat. Here's a healthy version that I can indulge in without too much guilt.

1 cup yellow cornmeal	1 teaspoon salt
½ cup whole wheat flour	2 egg whites
½ cup quick oatmeal	1 cup plain nonfat yogurt
1 tablespoon raw brown sugar	1½ cups nonfat milk
1 tablespoon baking soda	Canola oil spray

Preheat griddle or large skillet to medium. The griddle is ready when a few drops of water "dance" on the griddle or skillet.

Combine the dry ingredients and mix well. Add the egg whites, yogurt, and milk and mix until combined. Add just the amount of milk you want to get the batter you desire. Thinner batter makes thinner pancakes, a thicker batter makes thicker pancakes.

Spray preheated griddle or skillet with canola oil spray. Working in batches, spoon 2 tablespoons batter onto griddle for each pancake. Cook until golden brown, about 2 minutes per side. You will need to re-spray canola oil on griddle after each batch, since there is no oil in these pancakes. Serve with *Fresh Fruit Compote*.

Serves 4

Fresh Fruit Compote

This is a nice healthy alternative to syrup for your pancakes or French toast. It's loaded with antioxidants, warm, inviting, and yummy!

1 cup fresh blueberries	1 teaspoon cinnamon
1 cup fresh strawberries, sliced	Juice of ½ lemon
1 banana, sliced	Canola oil spray
1 peach, diced	

Spray a medium sized skillet with canola oil spray, and place all ingredients in pan. Cook over a low heat until all of the ingredients meld together and the mixture thickens. Serve with *Cornmeal Pancakes, Oatmeal Pancakes*, or *Stuffed French Toast*.

Serves 4

Green Omelet

This omelet is so packed with cancer-fighting broccoli and spinach, I should've called it the antioxidant omelet! Not only does this make a beautiful presentation topped with salsa, but it tastes great too.

1 tablespoon canola oil
1 cup broccoli, chopped finely
1 bunch scallions, chopped
5 egg whites + 2 whole eggs
¼ cup nonfat milk

1 cup spinach, chopped
¼ cup flat-leaf parsley, chopped
Canola oil spray
½ cup salsa to garnish (optional)

Pour canola oil into a small skillet and allow to heat up over a medium heat. Place broccoli and scallions in skillet and sauté for 4-5 minutes until scallions begin to turn translucent. Remove from heat.

Whisk together egg whites, eggs, and milk. Spray a medium skillet with canola oil spray and place over a low heat. Pour in eggs. After about 1 minute, when the eggs begin to cook, layer in vegetables on one side of the pan. Continue cooking on a very low heat and cover with a tight lid. This will allow the eggs to get puffy. When fully cooked, flip the side of the omelet without the filling over onto the side with the filling. Remove from heat. Serve topped with salsa or with a side of sliced tomatoes.

Serves 2

Indian Spiced Egg Scramble

Here's a twist on a traditional egg scramble. Currently being looked at in many studies, the spice turmeric is believed by some researchers to prevent and slow the growth of a number of different types of cancer.

1 medium unpeeled potato, finely diced
1 medium onion, finely diced
1 cup fresh spinach, chopped
2 medium tomatoes, diced
6 egg whites

½ teaspoon curry
½ teaspoon turmeric
¼ teaspoon cumin
1 tablespoon cilantro, chopped
Canola oil spray

Spray a medium skillet generously with canola oil spray, and add potato and onion. Sauté until potatoes brown and onions are translucent (about 10 minutes). Add spinach and tomatoes, stir until spinach wilts. In a medium bowl, whisk together the egg whites, curry, turmeric, and cumin. Add to skillet, mix well. Cook on a low heat until eggs are fully cooked. Top with fresh cilantro. Serve warm.

Serves 2

Hash Brown Egg Casserole

I don't eat eggs often, but this is a semi-healthy version of an otherwise fat-laden original. Egg casseroles are usually loaded with fat from cheese and sausages. I use mostly egg whites and low-fat cheese. This is not a dish to eat every weekend, but it's a nice dish to share with company because it can be prepared the day before, covered with plastic wrap, and cooked the next morning. My guests always want the recipe before they leave!

2 tablespoons canola oil
1 large onion, diced
1 green pepper, chopped
1 red pepper, chopped
2 cups shredded, unpeeled, white potatoes
2 cups shredded, peeled, sweet potatoes

4 eggs + 12 egg whites
1 cup nonfat milk
¼ cup chopped flat-leaf parsley
1 cup shredded cheese (part-skim mozzarella, veggie, or soy)
¼ cup low-fat grated Parmesan cheese
Canola oil spray
Salt and pepper

Preheat oven to 350 degrees F. Pat the shredded potatoes dry with a paper towel.

Heat the canola oil in a large skillet and add the oil, onion, green pepper, and red pepper. Sauté until vegetables are soft. Set aside.

Spray a large skillet or griddle generously with canola oil spray. Add both types of shredded potatoes. Salt and pepper the potatoes as they are cooking. Cook for 10 minutes over a medium heat, and then turn the potatoes over for another 10 minutes. When they are soft, set aside.

Whisk together the whole eggs, egg whites, and milk. Stir in the parsley.

Spray a 9" x 13" baking dish with canola oil spray. Spread the hash browns over the bottom of the pan. Layer the cooked onion and peppers over the potatoes. Sprinkle the shredded cheese on top of the vegetables. Pour the egg mixture over the top, covering the entire casserole. Sprinkle Parmesan cheese over the top.

Cover with aluminum foil and cook in the preheated oven for 45 minutes. Remove the foil and cook for another 15 minutes or until set. Serve immediately.

Serves 6-8

Oatmeal Pancakes

These pancakes are guilt free because they're made without the customary fats and sugars. Once you've enjoyed these a few times, you might not even want the traditional kind!

1½ cups nonfat or soy milk
½ teaspoon vinegar
1 cup white whole wheat flour
1 cup old-fashioned oatmeal
1 tablespoon raw brown sugar

1 teaspoon baking soda
¼ teaspoon salt
2 large egg whites, lightly beaten
1 cup plain nonfat yogurt
Canola oil spray

Preheat griddle or large skillet to medium-high. It's ready when a few drops of water sprinkled on the surface dance. Pour the vinegar into the milk to make a faux buttermilk. Set aside.

In a large bowl, combine flour, oatmeal, sugar, baking soda, and salt. In a smaller bowl, combine egg whites, faux buttermilk, and yogurt. Pour the wet ingredients into the dry ingredients, and mix well.

Spray the preheated griddle or skillet with canola oil spray. Immediately, so the oil doesn't burn, and working in batches, spoon 2 tablespoons batter onto griddle or skillet for each pancake. Cook until golden brown, about 2 minutes per side. You will need to re-spray canola oil on griddle or skillet after each batch, since there is no oil in these pancakes. Serve with *Fresh Fruit Compote*.

Serves 3-4

Whole Grain Hot Cereal

To make your hurried mornings easier, make a week in bulk and store it in the refrigerator.

4 cups water
½ cup whole grain wheat, cracked
½ cup steel cut oats

1 teaspoon cinnamon
¼ cup raisins

In a large saucepan, bring the water to a boil. Stir in the oats, wheat, and cinnamon. Cover and lower the heat to a simmer. Continue to simmer for 20-30 minutes, or until water is absorbed and grain is the desired consistency. Add the raisins and stir well. Remove from heat and serve immediately, or allow to cool and store in an airtight container in the refrigerator. Reheat before serving.

Note: Add a little water to thin it out when reheating.

Makes 6-8 servings

Ricotta Blueberry Pancakes

This is a nice, special, Sunday morning breakfast, great to serve guests. The pancakes are nice and fluffy, and the blueberries are hot and juicy. In addition to helping to make these pancakes a tasty treat, new studies show that blueberries help inhibit cancer cells.

1 cup nonfat or soy milk
Juice of 1 lemon
1¼ cups white whole wheat flour
¼ cup quick oatmeal
1 teaspoon raw brown sugar
1 teaspoon baking powder
½ teaspoon baking soda
½ teaspoon nutmeg
½ teaspoon salt

¾ cup nonfat or part-skim ricotta cheese
Zest of 1 lemon
¼ cup orange juice
2 large egg whites
½ teaspoon vanilla
¾ cup fresh or frozen (unthawed) blueberries
Canola oil spray

Preheat oven to 250 degrees F. Squeeze lemon into milk to make a faux buttermilk. Set aside.

Preheat a griddle or large skillet to medium-high. The griddle, or skillet, is ready when you drop a few water droplets onto it, and the water dances.

Combine dry ingredients (flour, oatmeal, sugar, baking powder, baking soda, salt, and nutmeg) in a large bowl and mix well. In another bowl, combine ricotta, faux buttermilk, lemon zest, orange juice, egg whites, and vanilla. Whisk until well combined and frothy. Mix dry ingredients into the wet ingredients. Fold in the blueberries.

When the griddle or skillet is hot, spray with canola oil spray. Immediately, so the oil doesn't burn, spoon 1/4 cup of batter onto the griddle for each pancake. Cook until the bottom of the pancake is golden brown and bubbles appear on the top of the pancake. When the bubbles form, flip the pancakes and continue cooking on the other side for about 2-3 minutes more. Repeat, spraying the griddle with the canola oil spray for each new batch, until all the batter is used.

Place the cooked pancakes directly on your oven rack while the next batch cooks. These pancakes tend to be a little moist and the extra cooking in the oven, at the low temperature, dries them out to the perfect consistency. Serve hot with *Fresh Fruit Compote*.

Makes 18 pancakes

Stuffed French Toast

This is a rich, decadent treat that couldn't be easier to make. Years ago I used to frequent a small diner in Wichita, Kansas that served a deluxe peanut butter and jelly sandwich with bananas and nuts. This is my healthier version. The fruit inside the toast gets warm and gooey, and there's plenty of good stuff in here, too. Blueberries, walnuts, cinnamon, and almond butter are all full of antioxidants that help protect you against cancer.

4 pieces whole grain or whole wheat bread
4 tablespoons almond butter
2 bananas, sliced thinly long-ways
4 large strawberries, sliced thinly
½ cup fresh blueberries
2 eggs
1 cup nonfat or soy milk
1 teaspoon cinnamon
½ teaspoon salt
½ teaspoon almond extract
Zest of 1 large orange
Zest of 1 large lemon
¼ cup chopped walnuts, toasted
Dusting of powdered sugar (optional)
Canola oil spray

Spread almond butter evenly over 4 pieces of bread, as this will help hold the French toast together. Place the sliced bananas evenly on top of almond butter on 2 pieces of bread. Place sliced strawberries evenly on top of banana slices and blueberries evenly on top of strawberries.

Make 2 sandwiches by placing the almond butter covered pieces of bread on top of the fruit layered pieces of bread. Press the sandwiches down lightly so that they hold together when dipped into the egg mixture. Cut sandwich into quarters diagonally.

In a medium bowl, mix the egg, milk, cinnamon, salt, and almond extract, and whisk together well. Dip the sandwich quarters into the egg mixture to coat thoroughly.

Preheat a griddle or skillet to medium. When you are ready to place the French toast on the griddle or skillet, spray the preheated griddle or skillet with canola oil spray. Place the dipped sandwich quarters onto griddle or skillet and cook for 3 minutes on each side, flipping the sandwiches until both sides have a golden brown color.

When finished cooking, dust with zests and toasted walnuts. Dust with a very light dusting of powdered sugar, if desired. Serve with *Fresh Fruit Compote*.

Serves 2-3

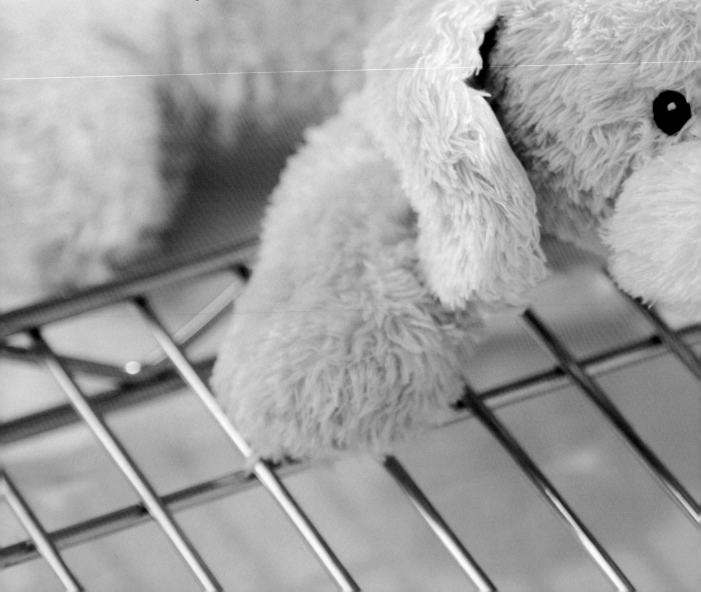

A package came in the mail shortly after my diagnosis. In it was a soft little blue stuffed dog. It was sent from an acquaintance, someone I had only met a couple of times, but who had heard about my illness and wanted to express her support.

I was so touched that someone would take the time to send me this little guy that he became my mascot through my cancer journey. I call him Norm, short for Normal, because that's what I wanted, to get back to normal. Norm stuck by me all the way, giving his quiet support and unconditional love. He is still with me, and he supervised most of the cooking that went into creating this cookbook!

Smoothies and Snacks

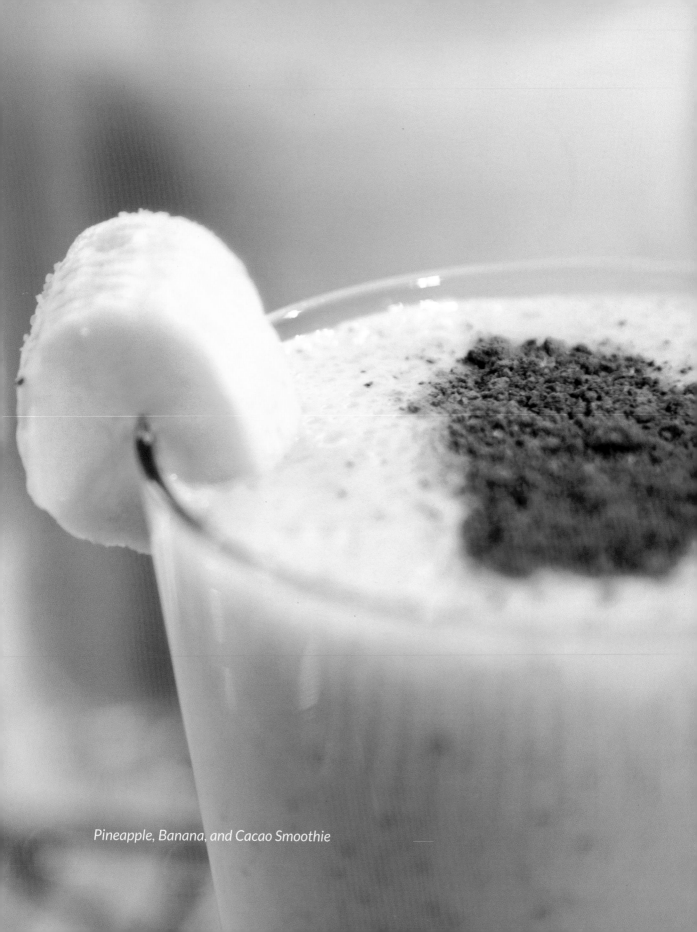

Pineapple, Banana, and Cacao Smoothie

Snacks, unfortunately, are often our modern day dietary downfall. We tend to love to fill up on things that are sugary, salty, and laden with refined and hydrogenated omega-6s (Foods to Avoid). It's time to change all that, to retrain our palates to enjoy healthier versions of between-meal goodies.

Most of the time, for a snack, I enjoy raw nuts like almonds or walnuts, or maybe some home-popped popcorn, prepared without butter or unhealthy oils. When I want something a little different, I turn to my new favorites like smoothies, frozen fruits, or roasted garbanzo beans.

Smoothies are such easy things to make. Just put some ingredients in the blender, add ice, rev it up, and you've got a great, frosty treat. Many smoothies, especially those bought at coffee shops, have hidden fat and sugars in them. The signs at the stores may say "healthy," but that's not always true.

These smoothie recipes are a few of my favorites, but smoothies can be a mix and match food. Whatever fruit or juice you have sitting in your refrigerator will probably make a tasty treat. Think of these recipes as a jumping off place. Start with my ideas, and use your imagination to blend up some liquid magic!

Almond Butter Smoothie

Almond butter is made from nothing but almonds, and as such is a nutritional powerhouse. Almonds are low in saturated fat (the bad stuff), high in monounsaturated fats (the good stuff), and they contain no transfat (the worst stuff). This smoothie tastes like a rich, decadent shake.

1 cup plain nonfat yogurt
1 cup nonfat, soy, or almond milk
1 banana, peeled, cut in chunks, and frozen
2 tablespoons almond butter

1 tablespoon maple syrup
½ teaspoon cinnamon
1 cup ice cubes

Place all of the ingredients in a blender and blend until smooth. **Serves 2**

Apricot Pineapple Smoothie

Apricots are excellent sources of Vitamins A and C and beta-carotene. The apricot is a little fruit that packs a big nutritional punch.

½ cup canned crushed pineapple, unsweetened
3 fresh apricots, pitted or 3 dried
2 large strawberries, tops removed

½ banana, peeled, cut in thirds, and frozen
1 cup plain nonfat yogurt
1 cup ice cubes

Place all of the ingredients in a blender and blend until smooth. **Serves 2**

Mango Smoothie

Mangoes contain several phytochemicals, are high in fiber, Vitamins, and are fat free. Mangoes also contain beta-carotene, and studies have shown that it can help reduce the risk of some cancers. Drink one of these and you'll feel like you're on a tropical vacation!

1 large orange, rind removed and seeded
1 fresh mango, peeled, sliced, and frozen
1 banana, peeled, cut in thirds, and frozen

1 cup plain nonfat yogurt
¾- 1 cup nonfat or soy milk

You'll need to freeze the mango and banana ahead of time for this smoothie. The frozen fruit will thicken the smoothie instead of using ice.

Place all of the ingredients in a blender and blend until smooth. Add the amount of milk needed to attain the consistency you desire. **Serves 2**

Banana Orange Smoothie

Bananas are sometimes called the perfect fruit, and they are certainly one of the most popular. They're high in fiber, potassium, and Vitamin C. Oranges are also high in Vitamin C, as well as being rich in calcium and beta-carotene, among other nutrients. This recipe is a simple, old-fashioned banana smoothie that will certainly satisfy on a hot summer's day. Sometimes simple is better.

1 banana, peeled and cut in thirds
1 large orange (or 2 small), peeled, seeded, and quartered

¼ cup orange juice
1 cup plain nonfat yogurt
1 cup ice cubes

Place all of the ingredients in a blender and blend until smooth. **Serves 2**

Berry Smoothie

Berries are considered by many to be a super food. Research has proven that berries have one of the highest antioxidant contents of all foods and they contain phytochemicals that help fight cancer.

1 cup fresh orange juice
1 cup plain nonfat yogurt
1 cup fresh strawberries

1 cup fresh blueberries
½ cup fresh raspberries
1 cup ice cubes

Place all of the ingredients in a blender and blend until smooth. **Serves 2**

Pineapple, Banana, and Cacao Smoothie

This is a wonderful, thick smoothie that tastes more like a chocolate shake. Just put any bananas that begin to get too ripe into the freezer and save them for when you want to make this shake. I open a can of pineapple, and split it into 2 plastic freezer bags, then freeze them so they're ready to go.

1 ripe banana, frozen
¾ cup frozen pineapple chunks, unsweetened (fresh, canned, or packaged)
1 cup plain nonfat yogurt
1 cup nonfat or soy milk

1 tablespoon unsweetened cacao powder
1 tablespoon maple syrup
1 teaspoon vanilla extract
4 ice cubes

Place all ingredients into a blender and blend until smooth. **Serves 2**

Kale Smoothie

Kale may seem strange in a smoothie, but it actually makes a great ingredient when mixed with frozen fruit. Kale has been shown to help boost your immune system and reduce the risk of many cancers. It's a fun way to get your cruciferous vegetables in!

1 banana, peeled, cut in thirds, and frozen
10 kale leaves, large vein down the middle removed
1 mango, peeled, cubed, and frozen

1 cup pineapple, peeled, cubed, and frozen
1 cup ice cubes
1 cup fresh orange juice
1 cup pure pineapple juice

Place all of the ingredients in a blender and blend until smooth. **Serves 2**

Roasted Garbanzo Beans

Garbanzo beans (chickpeas) are high in fiber, high in protein, and have been proven in studies to help prevent certain cancers. There are a lot of nutrients in these little beans. These beans are great as a snack all by themselves or may be served atop a crisp salad.

2 (15 ounce) cans garbanzo beans (chickpeas)
2 teaspoons cumin
2 teaspoons granulated garlic

1 teaspoon chili powder
4 teaspoons olive oil
Canola oil spray
Salt and pepper

Preheat oven to 375 degrees F. Drain garbanzo beans and rinse well with cold water. Dry beans with a paper towel until no water is left and beans are totally dry.

In a medium-size mixing bowl, toss garbanzo beans with olive oil and spices. Spray baking sheet with canola oil spray. Arrange in a single layer on baking sheet. Bake until they are slightly browned and crisp, about 45 minutes, stirring occasionally.

Sprinkle with salt and pepper if desired.

Serves 3-4

Peach Smoothie

Peaches are called stone fruits because of their pits. Stone fruits are rich in phenols (organic compounds) and these phenols have shown promising results in laboratory tests fighting breast cancer cells.

2 peaches, pitted, in chunks, and frozen
1 cup plain nonfat yogurt
½ cup fresh orange juice

½ cup nonfat or soy milk
1 tablespoon maple syrup
1 cup ice cubes

Place all of the ingredients in a blender and blend until smooth. **Serves 2**

Healthy Trail Mix

Making your own trail mix is super simple and better than store bought. Moderation is to be used here. Even though the ingredients are healthy, nuts and dark chocolate are high in calories. Maintaining a healthy weight is extremely important for cancer prevention.

½ cup quick oats
1 teaspoon cinnamon
Canola oil spray
½ cup raw almonds
½ cup raw walnuts

½ cup pecans
½ cup raisins
½ cup raw sunflower seed kernels
2 ounces dark chocolate,
70% or more cacao, ¼ inch pieces

Preheat oven to 350 degrees F. In a small bowl, combine cinnamon and quick oats. Spray oats with canola oil spray to help cinnamon stick to oats. Mix well. Spread oats evenly over a cookie sheet. Spread almonds and walnuts evenly over another cookie sheet. Place both cookie sheets into preheated oven for 10-15 minutes to toast. Be careful not to burn. Remove from oven. Allow to cool for 1 minute.

Place oats, almonds, and walnuts in a medium bowl. Add pecans, raisins, and sunflower seed kernels. Mix together well. Add chocolate last and mix well again. Chocolate will melt a little because the nuts will still be hot from the oven, and small, tasty clusters will form. Spread mixture evenly over one of the cookie sheets and place in the refrigerator until the chocolate hardens. Once the chocolate hardens, it can be removed the refrigerator.

Makes 12 servings

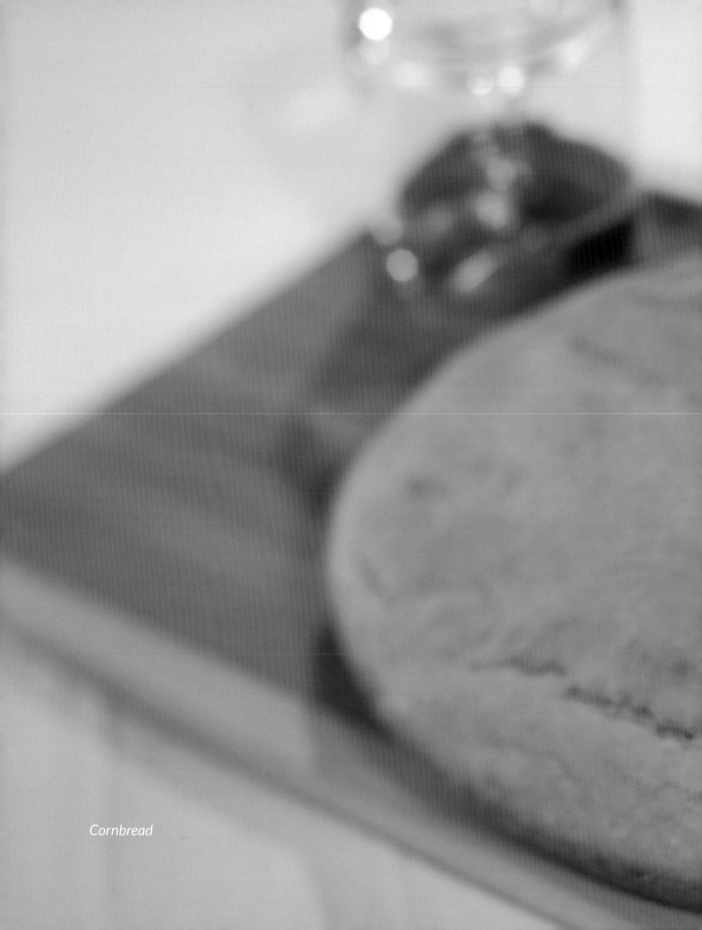

Cornbread

Breads

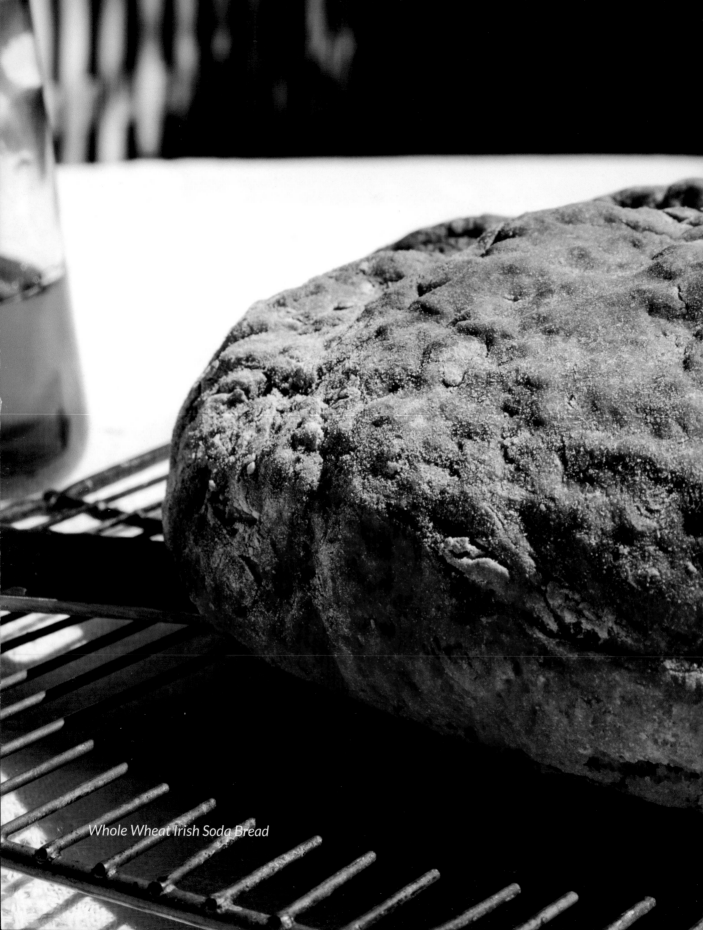

Whole Wheat Irish Soda Bread

Most of today's mass-produced, processed breads are depleted of nutrients and include unnecessary chemicals and additives. Next time you go to the store, check out a Nutrition Facts label on a loaf of bread. The bread will probably contain high fructose corn syrup, other sugars, and myriad chemicals All of that is in your bread and will be going into your body. No thanks!

If you do decide to buy your bread instead of bake it yourself, start reading the labels. Many of the new "artisan" breads are made with minimal ingredients, including whole grains, and are intended to be purchased and eaten right away, not processed to sit on a shelf for days.

The best way to avoid unnecessary ingredients and additives is to try to make your own bread when time permits. Making bread is simple and really doesn't take that much actual work. Yes, there is a waiting period if you're working with a yeast dough, but the labor itself is minimal.

The breads in this section are made with flours other than white, and with little or no vegetable oils or butter. Some are snack breads, some are sandwich breads, and some are good as a side to a meal. Please note that these breads are not on the sweet side, even the coffee cake breads. Sugars are in my Foods to Avoid section, so I have used them minimally or not at all. As I stated in the Introduction, the more you refrain from eating the sugary sweet foods, the more you won't desire them.

Note that even though the breads are baked with healthier ingredients, calories still need to be considered. The Second Expert Report published by the American Institute for Cancer Research and The World Cancer Research Fund, clearly states that there is convincing evidence that body fat increases risk for certain cancers. They recommend maintaining a healthy body weight. That being said, there's no reason to totally avoid breads. Moderation is key.

I use a white whole wheat flour for my bread recipes. It is not milled from a red wheat, but rather a white spring wheat. It more closely resembles the texture of traditional all-purpose white flour. However, it does not have the bran and germ removed as white flour does, so it is still loaded with nutrients. Nowadays it should be readily found in your local supermarket.

Let's get back to bread being the "staff of life," and not the "shaft of life."

Apple, Carrot, and Raisin Muffins

This muffin recipe doesn't use any unhealthy fats. It gets its moisture from the applesauce and yogurt. Some studies have shown that diets high in fat increase the risk of cancer.

2 cups white whole wheat flour
1 cup quick oatmeal
1 cup oat or wheat bran
1 tablespoon baking soda
1 teaspoon ground cinnamon
1 teaspoon nutmeg
½ teaspoon ground cloves
1 teaspoon salt

1 large carrot, grated
2 apples, peeled and diced finely
1 cup raisins
1¼ cup unsweetened applesauce
1 cup plain nonfat yogurt
2 egg whites
1 teaspoon vanilla
Canola oil spray

Preheat oven to 375 degrees F. Combine flour, oatmeal, bran, baking soda, spices, and salt. Stir in carrots, apples, and raisins. Stir in applesauce, yogurt, egg whites, and vanilla until blended well.

Spray two standard 12-cup muffin pans with canola oil spray, and then fill cups ¾ full. Bake in preheated oven 20 to 23 minutes, or until knife inserted in center comes out clean. Cool in pan on wire rack 5 minutes. Remove muffins and cool slightly. Serve warm.

Makes 24 muffins

Cinnamon Banana Bread

Cinnamon, that innocuous little spice in your kitchen cabinet, can help regulate your blood sugar, lower your cholesterol, and (in a recent study) reduced the growth of leukemia and lymphoma cancer cells. Besides, who among us can resist the smell of fresh cinnamon bread baking on a Sunday morning?

2 cups white whole wheat flour
1 tablespoon raw brown sugar
¼ cup wheat germ
½ teaspoon salt
1 tablespoon baking powder
¼ teaspoon baking soda
2 egg whites
1 tablespoon cinnamon

½ cup plain nonfat yogurt
1 ripe banana, mashed
¾ cup skim milk
¼ cup canola oil
⅓ cup raisins
⅓ cup walnuts
Canola oil spray

Ciabatta Bread

3 cups wheat bread flour
1 cup unbleached flour
2 cups water (110-115 degrees F.)
1 package active dry yeast

1 teaspoon salt
1 tablespoon raw sugar
Flour for dusting
Canola oil spray

Dissolve yeast into ½ cup of warm water and allow to sit for 10 minutes.

Mix all other ingredients together (include 1½ cups warm water) and then add the yeast mixture. Stir until the mixture becomes a smooth yet sticky dough. Roll into a ball. Spray a clean surface with canola oil spray and knead the ball of dough on it until the dough is smooth, about 5 minutes. Add a small dusting of flour if necessary in kneading.

Spray a medium-sized bowl with canola oil spray and place dough in bowl. Cover with plastic wrap and set aside until dough doubles in size, about 1 hour.

Empty contents of bowl onto a floured, smooth surface. Cut dough in half and form into two 10 inch loaves. Place loaves on a greased baking sheet, leaving at least 4 inches between them. Cover lightly with plastic wrap and allow to rise until doubled in size (about 1 hour).

Preheat oven to 450 degrees F. Spray the loaves with water. Bake for 20-25 minutes.

Makes 2 loaves

Preheat oven to 350 degrees F.

In a large bowl, combine the dry ingredients (flour, sugar, wheat germ, salt, baking powder, baking soda, cinnamon) and mix well.

In a small bowl, combine the wet ingredients (egg whites, skim milk, oil, and yogurt), and whisk well. Whisk in the banana and combine well.

Add the wet ingredients to the dry ingredients. Stir in the raisins and the walnuts and mix well.

Spray a 9"x 5" loaf pan with canola oil spray. Pour the batter into the loaf pan. Bake for 40-45 minutes until top is golden and the bread sounds hollow when tapped. Allow bread to cool before removing from pan.

Makes 1 loaf

Citrus Poppy Seed Coffee Cake

This mid-morning snack is made with nonfat yogurt, which provides the moisture in the cake without the fat. It's not too sweet, yet it's satisfying and won't leave you hungry an hour later.

3 cups white whole wheat flour
1 cup quick oatmeal
1 tablespoon baking powder
1 teaspoon baking soda
½ cup raw brown sugar
3 tablespoons poppy seeds
2 egg whites

1 cup nonfat or soy milk
1 orange, zest and juice
1 lemon, zest and juice
Juice of 1 lime
1 cup plain nonfat yogurt
1 teaspoon salt
Canola oil spray

Preheat oven to 375 degrees F.

In a large bowl, combine flour, oatmeal, baking powder, baking soda, brown sugar, and poppy seeds (leave out 1 tablespoon poppy seeds and 1 tablespoon brown sugar) and mix well. Combine egg whites, milk, lemon (zest and juice), orange (zest and juice), lime juice, and yogurt in another bowl and whisk all together. Combine wet and dry ingredients and mix well.

Spray a 9" square cake pan with canola oil spray and fill with coffee cake batter. Sprinkle the remaining poppy seeds and brown sugar on top. Bake in preheated oven 45-50 minutes or until it tests done with a toothpick. This coffee cake freezes great and I like it for a nourishing mid-morning snack.

Makes 16-20 servings

Cornbread

1 cup cornmeal
1 cup white whole wheat flour
1 tablespoon baking powder
1 teaspoon salt
¾ cup nonfat milk

2 egg whites
2 tablespoons honey
½ cup *Yogurt Cheese*
2 tablespoons canola oil
Canola oil spray

Preheat oven to 400 degrees F. In a large bowl, combine dry ingredients. In a smaller bowl, mix together wet ingredients. Mix wet ingredients into dry ingredients until well blended. Spray an 8" square pan with canola oil spray and pour in bread batter. Place in preheated oven and bake for about 20 minutes or until done.

Makes 1 loaf

Garlic Bread

At one time, I made garlic bread with butter and tons of oil, but this is a much healthier version of that bread. It's simple and it works.

1 whole grain baguette
¼ cup olive oil

4 cloves garlic, minced
Salt and pepper

Preheat oven to 400 degrees F. Slice bread down the center lengthwise. Cut into 4 inch segments. Mix olive oil and garlic. Brush lightly with olive oil and garlic. Salt and pepper to taste. Place in oven directly on rack for 5 minutes, or until bread is slightly crunchy.

Serves 5-6

Plain Ol' Whole Wheat Bread

This bread has a nice crisp crust and is good for sandwiches or for a slice of toast in the morning.

1 package active dry yeast
½-1 cup water (110-115 degrees F.)
3¼ cups white whole wheat flour
1 teaspoon salt
1 tablespoon honey

½ cup nonfat milk (110-115 degrees F.)
2 tablespoons canola oil
Flour for dusting
Canola oil spray

Dissolve yeast into ½ cup warm water and allow to sit for 10 minutes.

In a large bowl combine flour and salt, stir to mix ingredients well. Add the honey, milk, yeast mixture, oil, and mix until all ingredients are incorporated. Dough will be lumpy and not smooth. Add the remaining water if necessary (dough should not be sticky.)

Turn out onto a clean, dry, floured surface and knead for 5 minutes or until dough is smooth. Place in a greased bowl and cover with plastic wrap. Allow to rise in a warm space until it doubles in size, about 1 hour.

Preheat oven to 375 degrees F. Punch the dough down and turn out again onto working surface. Shape into a roll and place into a 9" x 5" loaf pan sprayed with canola oil spray. Allow to rise until double again (about 1 hour).

Bake in preheated oven for 30 minutes. Remove from oven and carefully remove the bread from the pan. Cool on a rack.

Makes 1 loaf

Not So Flat Garlic Flatbread

These small breads make for a fun sandwich or dipping bread and are best served warm and toasty right off the grill.

1 package active dry yeast
1 cup water (110-115 degrees F.)
4 cups white whole wheat flour
½ cup nonfat milk, room temp.
2 egg whites
3 tablespoons raw brown sugar
1 teaspoon salt

4 cloves garlic, minced
½ cup nonfat milk (110-115 degrees F.)
¼ cup light olive oil
Flour for dusting
Canola oil spray
Salt and pepper

Dissolve yeast in a small bowl with water and allow to sit for 10 minutes.

In a large bowl, mix flour, milk, egg whites, sugar, and salt. Pour in yeast mixture and mix until a soft dough forms. Turn out of bowl and knead on a lightly floured surface for 5 minutes or until smooth.

Spray a large bowl with canola oil spray and place dough in the bowl. Cover with plastic wrap, and allow the dough to rise until it doubles in volume.

Punch down dough and knead in 3 cloves of the garlic. Divide into 12 pieces and roll into 12 small balls. Spray a cookie sheet with canola oil spray and place the balls on the cookie sheet. Cover with plastic wrap and allow to rise again until double.

Add the remaining garlic into the olive oil.

Preheat grill or a griddle to medium.

Once dough has risen for a second time, roll each ball out into a 5 inch circle with a rolling pin.

Place dough on grill or griddle and cook for 2-3 minutes until dough puffs up. Brush uncooked side with garlic olive oil and then turn the dough over. Brush the cooked side with the olive oil and cook until done, about 2-3 more minutes. Cook the remaining dough in the same manner. Serve hot off the grill for optimum flavor! Salt and pepper to taste.

Makes 12 flatbreads

Herb Bread

This bread is a little more work to prepare and takes a little more time, as it is a yeast bread, but it's well worth the time and trouble. Surprising though it may be, herbs, both dried and fresh, are loaded with powerful antioxidants.

1 package active dry yeast
¼ cup water (110-115 degrees F.)
1 tablespoon raw brown sugar
1½ cups nonfat milk, scalded and cooled to room temperature
½ cup light olive oil or canola oil
1 teaspoon salt
1 egg white
4½-5 cups white whole wheat flour

1 teaspoon minced garlic
½ teaspoon black pepper
1 teaspoon ground sage
1 teaspoon chopped fresh thyme
1 teaspoon chopped fresh rosemary
1 tablespoon chopped flat-leaf parsley
Flour for dusting
Canola oil spray

Preheat oven to 375 degrees F. Dissolve yeast into warm water and allow to sit for 10 minutes.

Add the sugar, milk, oil, salt, egg white, and 2 cups of the flour to the yeast mixture. Mix well with large spoon and cover with plastic wrap. Dough will be loose. Let rise in a warm place until bubbly, about 1 hour.

Add the garlic, pepper, and all of the herbs to the dough. Add the remaining flour until you have a smooth dough. You might need a little less or a little more flour depending on altitude. Remove dough from bowl and place on a clean, dry, floured surface. Knead for about 10 minutes until all ingredients are incorporated into a smooth dough. Roll into large ball. Place the ball of dough in a large, canola oil-sprayed bowl, cover with plastic wrap, and allow to rise again until doubled, about 1 hour.

Spray a 9" loaf pan with canola oil spray to grease it well.

Punch dough down and place in the greased loaf pan. Let rise until doubled again, about 1 hour. Bake in preheated oven for 40 minutes or until done. Remove bread from pan (carefully, pan will be hot) and cool on a rack.

Makes 1 loaf

Pumpkin Bread with Oatmeal Topping

Pumpkin is chock full of an important antioxidant, beta-carotene. Recent research indicates that a diet rich in foods that contain beta-carotene may reduce the risk of developing certain types of cancer. Besides, pumpkin bread baking is always a welcome smell in the kitchen.

1½ cups white whole wheat flour
¼ cup raw brown sugar
¼ cup quick oats
2 teaspoons baking powder
½ teaspoon cinnamon
½ teaspoon nutmeg
½ teaspoon cloves
½ teaspoon salt
½ cup nonfat milk

1 teaspoon lemon juice
1 cup canned pumpkin, plain
2 egg whites
¼ cup unsweetened applesauce
¼ cup canola oil
¼ cup raisins
Canola oil spray
½ cup chopped walnuts

Preheat oven to 350 degrees F. Spray a 9" x 5" loaf pan with canola oil spray.

Add the lemon juice to the milk to make a faux buttermilk.

In a small bowl, mix dry ingredients together.

In a larger bowl, mix wet ingredients until well blended.

Combine the dry ingredients with the wet ingredients and stir until blended. Fold in the walnuts and raisins.

Pour into the prepared loaf pan.

Sprinkle *Oatmeal Topping* over the top of the loaf. Lightly press the topping into the loaf. Bake for 1 hour in the preheated oven or until golden brown.

Makes 1 loaf.

Oatmeal Topping

1 teaspoon canola oil
1 teaspoon raw brown sugar
¼ cup quick oats

1 teaspoon cinnamon
½ teaspoon ground cloves

Mix all ingredients until blended.

Sweet Potato Bread with Oatmeal Topping

Sweet potatoes are rich in complex carbohydrates, low in calories, and are a good source of fiber. They have been shown to help prevent both cancer and heart disease, and a four-ounce serving of sweet potato gives you half of your recommended daily allowance of Vitamin C. Sweet potatoes are more than just a holiday favorite, they are one of the most nutritious foods you can eat.

1 package active dry yeast
¼ cup water (110-115 degrees F.)
½ cup unsweetened apple juice
1¼ cups sweet potato, cooked and mashed

2 cups white whole wheat flour
¼ cup walnuts, chopped
1 teaspoon salt
Canola oil spray

Preheat oven to 350 degrees F. Dissolve yeast into warm water and allow to sit for 10 minutes.

In a large bowl, mix together all ingredients, including yeast mixture, except walnuts and ¼ cup whole wheat flour (for kneading). Mix well, until dough begins to form. Place dough on smooth, floured surface and knead for about 10 minutes. Add the remaining ¼ cup flour, as needed, until the dough is smooth and not sticky. Spray a bowl with canola oil spray and place the dough in the greased bowl. Cover with plastic wrap and set in a warm place until dough doubles in size, about 1 hour.

Spray a 9" x 5" loaf pan with canola oil spray. Punch the dough down, remove from bowl and place into the loaf pan to form a uniform loaf. Cover with plastic wrap and allow to rise again in a warm place for about an hour or until dough doubles.

Sprinkle *Oatmeal Topping* over the dough. Press the topping very lightly into the top of the dough. Place the bread into the preheated oven. Bake for about 30-35 minutes or until golden brown.

Makes 1 loaf

Whole Wheat Blueberry Muffins

Blueberries are a powerhouse of nutrients wrapped up in one small colorful package! Blueberries have natural compounds that probably prevent cancer and help with memory loss.

2 cups white whole wheat flour
1 tablespoon baking powder
½ teaspoon salt
2 tablespoons raw brown sugar
Zest of one lemon
Juice of one lemon
¾ cup milk

½ cup plain nonfat yogurt
1 ripe banana, mashed
2 egg whites
¼ cup canola oil
1 cup blueberries, fresh or frozen
Canola oil spray

Preheat oven to 350 degrees F. In a large bowl, mix together the dry ingredients. Add lemon zest to the dry ingredients. Then add lemon juice to the milk to make a faux buttermilk.

In a smaller bowl, mix together the wet ingredients. Whisk to blend well. Stir liquid ingredients into dry ingredients and mix well. Gently fold in the blueberries. Spray a 12-muffin tin with canola oil spray. Spoon muffin mixture into muffin tin and bake in preheated oven for 20 to 25 minutes or until golden.

Makes 12 muffins

Whole Wheat Irish Soda Bread

This is a nice, chewy bread that is satisfying with soups or stews on an autumn or winter night.

3 cups white whole wheat flour
1 cup all-purpose flour
1 teaspoon salt
2 teaspoons baking soda
2 teaspoons cream of tartar

1 tablespoon raw brown sugar
1½ cups skim milk
1 teaspoon vinegar
2 tablespoons olive oil
Flour for dusting

Preheat oven to 375 degrees F. Mix all dry ingredients in bowl. Make faux buttermilk by stirring vinegar into skim milk. Pour faux buttermilk into dry mixture. Add oil. Mix until dough is soft and pliable. Add more milk, if necessary. Dough should be moist, but not sticky. Shape into a flat circle (about 2 inches thick) on a lightly floured surface. Wet the blade of a sharp knife with water and cut a cross into the top of the dough. Place on a greased baking sheet and bake in a preheated oven for 40-45 minutes or until the crust is golden and the bread sounds hollow when tapped.

Makes 1 loaf

Whole Wheat Pita Bread

These breads are fun to make if you have the time. Also, if you've got kids—making bread with little pockets, what could be better? It's a quick, easy bread recipe and you don't have to worry about the preservatives or unhealthy oils that you might get in a store bought product. Pitas freeze beautifully, so make up a couple of batches and have them on hand to use for dipping or for a quick lunch!

1 cup + 2 tablespoons water (110-115 degrees F.)
1 package active dry yeast
1 tablespoon raw brown sugar
1 cup unbleached flour

2 cups white whole wheat flour
1½ teaspoons salt
1 tablespoon olive oil
Flour for dusting
Canola oil spray

Dissolve yeast and sugar in a small bowl with warm water and allow to sit for 10 minutes.

Place the flours and salt in a large bowl and add the yeast mixture along with the olive oil. Stir until flour and liquid make a moist dough.

Spray a clean, dry surface with canola oil spray and turn the dough onto the surface. Spray hands with canola oil spray also, to avoid dough sticking to your hands. Knead for 5 minutes, or until dough is smooth and not sticky to the touch. Sprinkle on extra flour if necessary.

Spray a large bowl with canola oil spray and place the dough in the bowl. Cover with plastic wrap and let stand in a warm place for about 1 hour or until dough has doubled in size. While dough is rising, preheat oven to 450 degrees F.

Punch down the dough and divide into 8 equal pieces. On a floured surface, roll out each piece to about 6 inch circles.

Spray a baking sheet with canola oil and place rounds on the sheet. Bake in the preheated oven for about 6 minutes until dough "puffs." Remove from oven and cooking sheet and wrap in a clean, dry towel to stay moist and soften. Press down gently on the towel to release the air in the pocket. When they are cool, you can slice them in half and use the pocket for filling. Place in a food storage bag to keep them moist.

Makes 8 pitas

Zucchini Bread

Zucchini is high in Vitamins A and C, both powerful antioxidants. The consumption of zucchini has also been proven in laboratories to be beneficial in fighting lung cancer. Besides, zucchini bread is an American classic! This whole wheat version is low-fat and uses a small amount of honey instead of a large amount of white sugar.

2 cups white whole wheat flour
1½ cups zucchini, finely shredded and packed
½ cup unsweetened applesauce
2 egg whites
¼ cup canola oil
3 tablespoons honey
1 teaspoon vanilla extract
1 teaspoon baking soda

1 teaspoon baking powder
1 tablespoon cinnamon
1 teaspoon nutmeg
½ teaspoon ground cloves
½ teaspoon salt
½ cup chopped walnuts
½ cup raisins
Canola oil spray

Preheat oven to 350 degrees F.

In a large bowl, combine the wet ingredients.

In another large bowl, combine the dry ingredients.

Combine wet and dry ingredients together and mix well. Fold in nuts and raisins.

Pour mixture into a canola oil-sprayed 9" x 5" loaf pan.

Bake in preheated oven for 1 hour or until done.

Remove bread from oven and cool on a wire rack.

Makes 1 loaf

Cinnamon Raisin Bread

Cinnamon is a spice most of us have in our cupboards and recently, in laboratory studies, it has shown to both inhibit the growth and spread of cancer. That's a lot of promise from one little spice.

2 cups white whole wheat flour
¼ cup raw brown sugar
½ teaspoon salt
1 tablespoon baking powder
1 teaspoon cinnamon
½ teaspoon nutmeg
1 teaspoon vinegar

1 cup nonfat milk
1 egg
2 tablespoons canola oil
½ cup raisins
½ cup chopped walnuts
Canola oil spray

Preheat oven to 350 degrees F.

In a large bowl combine flour, sugar, salt, baking powder, cinnamon, and nutmeg. Add vinegar to the milk to make a faux buttermilk. In a small bowl, whisk together the milk, egg, and oil.

Add the liquid mixture to the dry ingredients and stir to combine well. Stir in the raisins and ¼ cup walnuts.

Spray a 9"x 5" loaf pan with canola oil spray. Pour the batter into the loaf pan. Sprinkle the remaining ¼ cup chopped walnuts over the top of the batter. Press the walnuts lightly in the top of the batter. Bake for about 35 minutes until bread tests done. Allow bread to cool on a rack before removing from pan.

Note: You can substitute, for the topping, ¼ cup chopped Healthy Trail Mix for the last ¼ cup of chopped walnuts.

Makes 1 loaf

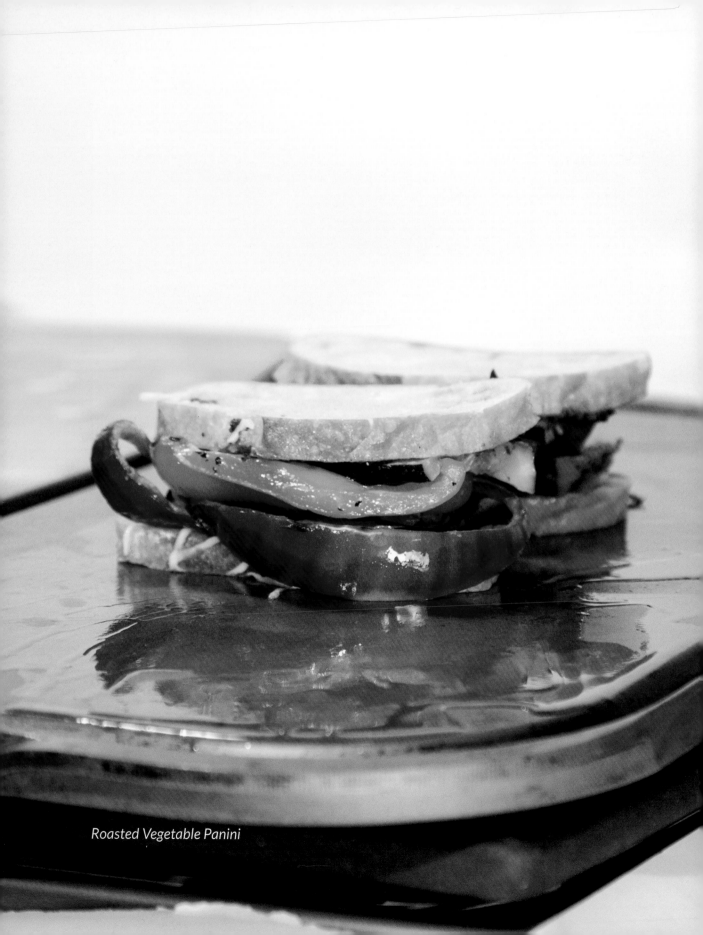

Roasted Vegetable Panini

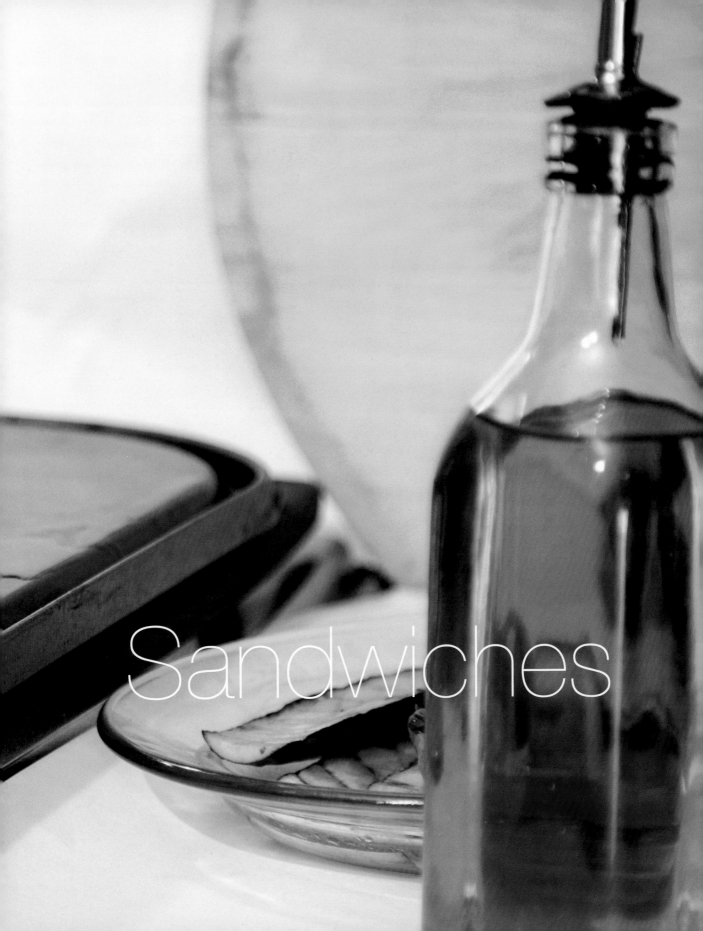

Sandwiches

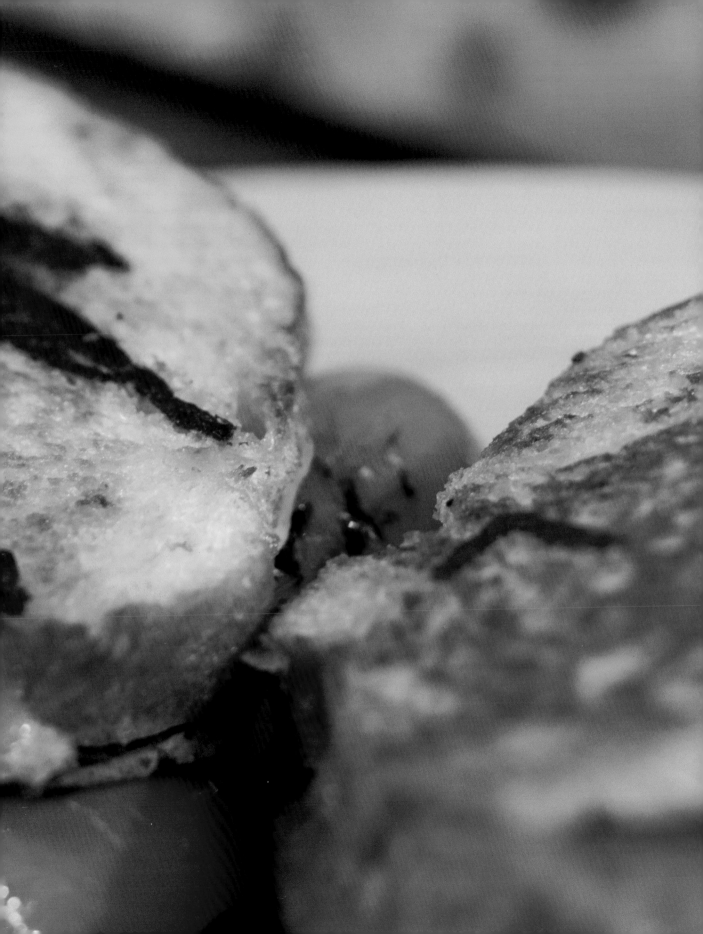

Sometimes you just want to stick something between two pieces of bread and chow down. Having a sandwich is okay, it's what we've gotten used to putting between those two pieces of bread that's the problem. Meats and fat-laden spreads are the usual problematic fare, with lunch-meat being the main culprit. According to the Second Expert Report published by the American Institute for Cancer Research and The World Cancer Research Fund, processed meats are some of the worst things we can eat with regard to trying to avoid cancer.

You can still enjoy a sandwich and stay healthy, you just have to choose the right ingredients to put between those two slices of whole grain bread! Serve up *Roasted Vegetable Panini*, for instance, at your next gathering and see if there are any complaints from the crowd.

Cheeseburger and Fries

I once had a vegetarian friend say to me, "I miss the burger experience." You won't with these! We love burger nights at my house. Although the burgers are great, the real treat on burger nights are these great fries as an accompaniment.

Mushroom Cheeseburgers

2 whole wheat buns
2 *Mushroom Veggie Burgers*

2 slices cheese (part-skim mozzarella, veggie, or soy)
Canola oil spray

Cook the burgers according to recipe directions, in a canola oil-sprayed skillet, placing a piece of cheese atop each patty the last minute of cooking. Serve with homemade fries and any of your favorite burger toppings such as avocado, grilled onions, hearty greens, or tomatoes.

Fries

1 large unpeeled russet potato
1 large peeled sweet potato or yam
2 tablespoons olive oil

Salt and pepper
Granulated garlic
Canola oil spray

Preheat oven to 450 degrees F. Pierce potatoes with a fork, and cook halfway through in the microwave. Microwave times vary—you don't want the potatoes totally cooked, just softened a little. That will cut the cooking time in the oven. Allow the potatoes to cool off from the microwave.

Slice the potatoes into French fry-size pieces. Place sliced potatoes in a bowl and drizzle with olive oil. Season to taste with salt, pepper, and garlic. Mix well. Place potatoes on a canola oil-sprayed cookie sheet so that they lay flat on the bottom of the sheet. Bake for about 15-30 minutes, turning potatoes with a spatula every 5 minutes or so to prevent burning. When brown and crispy, they are ready to eat!

Serves 2

Lavash Wraps

This is a fun sandwich to eat that's good for you too! Beans are, quite simply, a miracle food, and sprouts have shown in studies to help ward off certain cancers.

1 (12 inch) square of whole wheat lavash
½ cup *Hummus*
½ cup cucumber, seeded and diced
1 small onion, diced
1 medium tomato, seeded and diced
1 cup sprouts (any kind will do)

¼ cup shredded carrots
¼ cup red pepper, diced
½ teaspoon cumin
¼ cup chopped fresh cilantro
Salt and pepper

Spread the *Hummus* evenly on the lavash. Spread all other ingredients evenly over the *Hummus*. Roll the lavash up tightly into a long log and cut in half. Salt and pepper to taste. Serve cold.

Serves 2

Portobello Mushroom Burgers

Marinated portobello mushrooms make a great substitute for a hamburger. Tasty and meaty, they are low in fat, high in fiber, and have been known to exhibit anti-cancer properties. This is a good substitute for a summertime grilled favorite.

4 large portobello mushroom caps
½ cup balsamic vinegar
¼ cup extra-virgin olive oil
1 clove garlic, minced
2 tablespoons chopped fresh basil

2 tablespoons chopped flat-leaf parsley
4 slices part-skim mozzarella,
veggie, or soy cheese
4 whole wheat hamburger buns

Place all of the ingredients (except cheese and buns) into a quart-size plastic food storage bag and make sure the bag is closed well. Shake until well-mixed. Lay the bag out flat so that the mushrooms are lying flat, and place in the refrigerator to marinate at least 4 hours.

Remove contents from bag and place on a preheated grill or in a skillet. Cook for about 5 minutes on each side. Place cheese on top of mushroom during the last couple of minutes of cooking. Serve on a whole wheat bun with lettuce, tomato, pickles, all of your usual burger topping favorites.

Serves 4

Mushroom Veggie Burgers

These veggie burgers are easy to make and they taste great. They are much healthier for you than the ones you might buy in the store, and there is no chance of carcinogens when grilling. Make a double batch and store in the freezer for an easy "pop it on the grill" dinner.

Be creative with your toppings and you'll never miss the meat. Isn't that what makes a burger great, anyway? Try avocado, sweet or hot peppers, or arugula instead of lettuce. Your choice of toppings is only limited by your imagination!

2 tablespoons olive oil	1 egg
1 pound mushrooms, diced	1 tablespoon dehydrated onion
½ medium onion, diced	½ teaspoon celery salt
2 cloves garlic, minced	¼ teaspoon paprika
½ cup rolled oats	¼ teaspoon cracked black pepper
½ cup bread crumbs	¼ teaspoon celery seed
(preferably Panko)	¼ cup chopped flat-leaf parsley
½ cup shredded cheese (part-skim mozzarella, veggie, or soy)	Canola oil spray

Sauté the onions, garlic, and mushrooms in olive oil for about 5 minutes, until onions are soft and all of the water is out of the mushrooms. Set aside until cool enough to touch.

Mix together all other ingredients and add in the cooked onions, garlic, and mushrooms.

Stir until all ingredients are combined well and consistency resembles that of ground beef. Shape the mixture into 4 patties. Spray a skillet with canola oil spray and cook each patty until the burgers are done (about 5 minutes on each side). Be careful flipping the burgers, they tend to be a little crumbly and not as compacted as a meat burger.

Makes 4 burgers

Onion and Pepper Panini

I always loved an Italian pepper sandwich, and this is a great, relatively easy panini to make. Quick and easy, yet tasty and healthy!

¼ cup olive oil
1 large onion, sliced
1 large green pepper, seeded and sliced
1 large red pepper, seeded and sliced
1 clove garlic, minced

½ whole wheat baguette
6 fresh basil leaves
2 slices cheese (part-skim mozzarella, veggie, or soy)
Canola oil spray
Salt and pepper

If you have a panini grill, that's great. If not, cover an ordinary brick well with aluminum foil and use it to compress your panini.

In a large skillet, heat 2 tablespoons of the olive oil over medium heat. Add the onions, green pepper, red pepper, and garlic. Sauté the vegetables until tender. Salt and pepper to taste. Set aside.

Cut the bread into 2 sandwich portions and then cut the very top off of the bread so the top and bottom are both flat. Brush the bread, top and bottom, and the insides with the remaining olive oil.

Place on preheated griddle to lightly toast one side of the bread. The lightly toasted sides will be the inside of the sandwiches. Remove from griddle.

Layer the vegetables on the toasted sides of the 2 pieces of bread. Top with basil, cheese, and the tops of the bread. Place the sandwiches on the panini grill or on a griddle.

If using a panini grill, cook according to panini grill instructions until sandwich is cooked. If using the griddle, place the foil-covered brick on top of the sandwich. Cook for about 3 minutes and remove the brick. Flip the sandwich, replacing the foil-covered brick on top of the sandwich. Cook for another 3 minutes. Serve hot and enjoy!

Serves 2

Roasted Vegetable Panini

What better way to get your veggies?

¼ cup balsamic vinegar
¼ cup olive oil, plus olive
oil for brushing
1 clove garlic, minced
1 medium eggplant, sliced
lengthwise into ¼ inch strips
1 zucchini, sliced lengthwise
into ¼ inchstrips
4 medium portobello
mushrooms, sliced

1 medium onion, sliced into rings
1 whole wheat baguette
1 roasted red pepper, skin and seeds
removed (or jarred peppers)
4 tablespoons *Black Olive Tapenade*
4 slices part-skim mozzarella,
veggie, or soy cheese
Canola oil spray
Salt and pepper

If you have a panini grill, that's great. If not, cover an ordinary brick well with aluminum foil and use it to compress your panini.

Whisk together olive oil, balsamic vinegar, garlic, and salt and pepper. Place eggplant, zucchini, mushroom, and onion in a plastic bag along with the oil and vinegar marinade. Seal the bag tightly and place in the refrigerator for 1-3 hours.

If you have a panini grill, preheat to medium heat. Place marinated vegetables on the grill and cook until grill marks appear and vegetables are tender. Remove from grill and set aside. If you don't have a panini grill, you can grill your veggies on a outside grill or use your broiler, turning veggies to cook both sides. Remove from heat and set aside.

Cut the bread into 4 sandwich portions and then cut the very top off of the bread so the top and bottom of the bread are both flat. Brush the bread, top and bottom, and the insides with olive oil. Place on grill to lightly toast one side of the bread. The lightly toasted sides will be the inside of the sandwiches. Remove from grill.

Layer the vegetables on the toasted sides of 4 pieces of bread. Top with tapenade, cheese, and the top of the bread. Place the sandwiches on the panini grill or on a preheated griddle.

If using a panini grill, cook according to panini grill instructions until sandwich is cooked. If using the griddle, place the sandwiches on the canola oil-sprayed griddle and then place the foil-covered brick on top of the sandwich. Cook for about 3 minutes and remove the brick. Flip the sandwich, replacing the foil-covered brick on top of the sandwich. Cook for another 3 minutes. Serve hot and enjoy!

Serves 4

Salad Pitas

This is a quick and healthy lunch, and flexible, so it's a great way to get rid of salad leftovers. Just make a salad to your liking and stuff a pita with it! Easy, quick, and nutritious.

4 whole wheat pitas, cut in half
12 tablespoons *Hummus*
2 cups hearty greens, chopped
½ small cucumber, diced
1 large tomato, diced
½ cup cooked brown rice
1 large ripe avocado, diced

¼ cup balsamic vinegar
¼ cup olive oil
⅓ cup shredded cheese (part-skim mozzarella, veggie, or soy)
¼ cup chopped onion
Salt and pepper

Open up pitas and spread 3 tablespoons of the *Hummus* inside each pita. Place all other ingredients in a large bowl and mix well. Stuff pitas with your salad mixture. Top with shredded cheese.

Serves 4

Salmon Burgers

This one satisfies the burger urge without the fat of a regular burger and with the addition of omega-3s from the salmon. Omega-3s have been shown to help prevent cancer cell growth.

24 ounces wild salmon
¼ cup chopped flat-leaf parsley
¼ cup chopped fresh dill
1 tablespoon finely chopped chives
2 tablespoons Dijon mustard
Juice of 2 lemons

2 cloves garlic, minced
½ cup shredded cheese (part-skim mozzarella, veggie, or soy)
½ teaspoon salt
½ teaspoon pepper
Olive oil spray

Finely chop raw salmon either by hand or, preferably, in a food processor, until it looks like ground meat. Place salmon in a bowl with all other ingredients (except olive oil spray) and mix well. Form into 4 patties. Spray a skillet with olive oil spray and cook on a medium-low heat for 5 minutes. Flip once and heat on the other side for 2 minutes or until done. Cook slowly so burgers don't burn. For a fun, tasty treat, instead of lettuce and tomato alongside, serve with a big leaf of mustard greens and tomato! The mustard greens compliment the flavor of the Dijon mustard in the burgers perfectly.

Makes 4 burgers

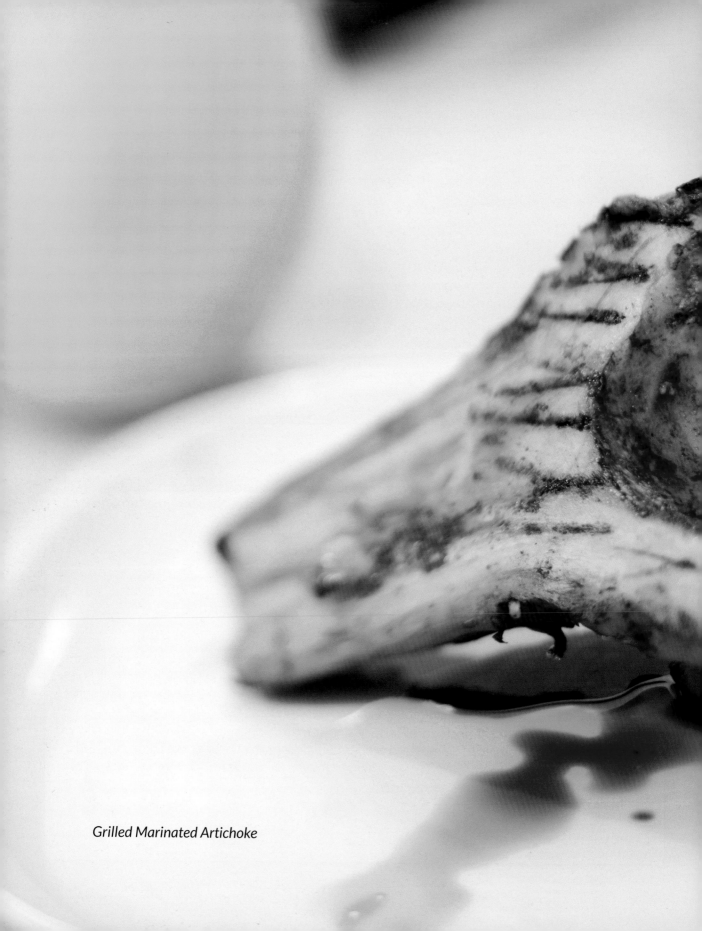

Grilled Marinated Artichoke

Dressings

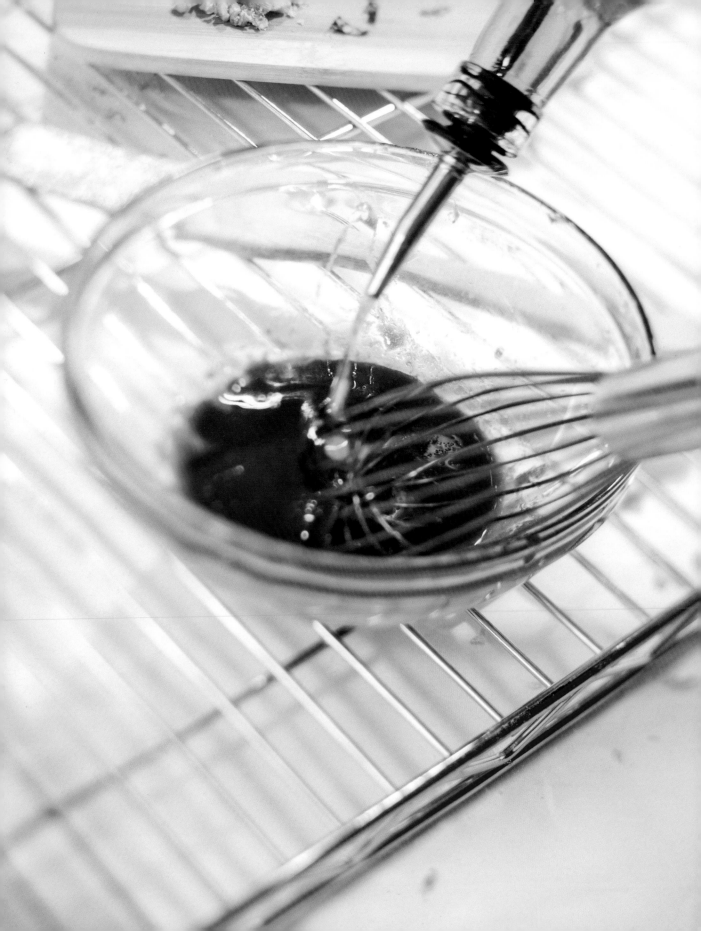

Making your own salad dressing is easy, and homemade dressing will be much healthier than what you can buy in the store. Take a look at a salad dressing label—just for laughs—you probably won't even be able to pronounce half the ingredients!

Most of the time I simply use balsamic vinegar and extra-virgin olive oil on my salads. Occasionally, I like to go the extra mile and make something special—especially when I have company coming over!

Making your own dressing gives you control over the ingredients. It tastes fresher and is fresher. All of my dressings contain extra-virgin olive oil, which is loaded with health benefits. Extra-virgin olive oil is rich in monounsaturated fats and contains the antioxidants Vitamin E, carotenoids, and oleuropein. The oil has to be cold-pressed. Extra-virgin olive oil, however, as that is the only olive oil that comes from pressing olives without the use of heat or chemicals. It contains phytochemicals that are otherwise lost in the refining process.

It might take a couple of extra minutes to blend up your own salad dressing, but it will be time well spent. We're worth it, and so is our health.

Asian Salad Dressing

Ginger not only tastes great but has also been proven in laboratory tests to help fight cancer cells. Studies pertaining to colon and ovarian cancer are still ongoing with this interesting, tasty root. Ginger has been shown to have antioxidant, anti-inflammatory, and anti-tumor properties. So why not use it whenever possible? This dressing is a fine way to "get your ginger."

⅓ cup red wine vinegar
¾ cup extra-virgin olive oil
2 tablespoons light soy sauce
3 cloves garlic, minced

2 tablespoons honey, warmed to thin it out a little bit
2 tablespoons fresh ginger root, minced
Dash of pepper

Whisk all ingredients together until smooth.

Creamy Cilantro Salad Dressing

Cilantro is a little herb with big possibilities. Coriander, the plant from which the flavorful herb leaves of cilantro come, is rich in phytonutrients and has long been known for its anti-inflammatory properties. When tested in lab experiments, coriander has been shown to lower blood sugar and cholesterol. Cilantro is a wonderful herb to add to your diet whenever possible.

½ cup extra-virgin olive oil
¼ cup cilantro, chopped finely
1 clove garlic, minced
3 scallions, chopped finely

2 tablespoons plain nonfat yogurt
1 tablespoon lime juice
Salt and pepper

Whisk all ingredients together until smooth. Serve chilled.

Creamy Tomato Salad Dressing

This is a healthier version of a fat-laden favorite. It has lots of good fresh herbs and lots of flavor.

½ cup *Yogurt Cheese*
1 large tomato, seeds removed and roughly chopped
2 tablespoons extra-virgin olive oil
2 tablespoons tomato paste
1 teaspoon Worcestershire sauce (organic, without high-fructose corn syrup)

1 tablespoon honey
1 tablespoon balsamic vinegar
1 clove garlic, minced
1 tablespoon minced fresh basil
1 teaspoon minced fresh oregano
Salt and pepper

Place all ingredients in a blender and blend until smooth. Serve chilled.

Honey Mustard Dressing

Prepared mustard is made from mustard seeds, which are part of the Brassica plant group, and are full of agents that have been found to prevent different types of cancer. Mustard is tangy, flavorful, and good for you to boot. Who knew?

2 tablespoons cider vinegar
3 tablespoons honey
1 cup plain nonfat yogurt
1 tablespoon Dijon mustard
1 teaspoon dry mustard

1 tablespoon red onion, chopped
2 tablespoons fresh flat-leaf parsley, chopped
Salt and pepper

Place all ingredients in a blender and blend until smooth. Serve chilled.

Hummus Salad Dressing

Hummus makes a great, thick basis for a salad dressing. Beans of all types, garbanzo included (which is what hummus is made from), are super healthy. I use *Hummus* in this recipe, but my *Black Bean Dip* would, as an option, also work perfectly in this dressing.

¼ cup *Hummus*
Juice of 1 lemon
2 tablespoons balsamic vinegar

2 tablespoons extra-virgin olive oil
Salt and pepper

Whisk together all ingredients until smooth.

Minced Herb Salad Dressing

This is a nice, multipurpose salad dressing that is loaded with antioxidant-rich, fresh herbs.

¼ cup minced fresh flat-leaf parsley
¼ cup minced fresh cilantro
1 teaspoon finely chopped fresh rosemary
3 cloves garlic, minced
2 tablespoons red wine vinegar

¼ cup extra-virgin olive oil
Juice of one lemon
Zest of ½ lemon
Salt and pepper

Whisk all ingredients together until smooth.

Roasted Garlic and Tomato Salad Dressing

Garlic is a powerful antioxidant, and roasted garlic has been found to help in the prevention of certain cancers of the digestive system.

1 head garlic	2 tablespoons fresh onion, minced
¼ cup + 1 tablespoon extra-virgin olive oil	¼ cup balsamic vinegar
2 large tomatoes, seeds removed and diced	2 tablespoons chopped fresh basil
Juice of 1 lemon	2 tablespoons chopped flat-leaf parsley
	Salt and pepper

Preheat oven to 400 degrees F. Roast garlic by cutting off the top of the garlic bulb, exposing the garlic cloves. Place bulb on a piece of aluminum foil that is large enough to wrap completely around the bulb. Drizzle 1 tablespoon of the olive oil over the garlic cloves. Wrap the foil around the garlic, making sure to close the foil tightly, and place into the preheated oven. Bake for 40 minutes.

Once garlic is finished roasting, remove from the oven and allow it to cool. Once cool, squeeze pulp out of the bulb and place in a blender along with all of the other ingredients. Blend until smooth.

Roasted Red Pepper Dressing with Herbs

Both red peppers and the herb basil have been shown to have potent antioxidants that help fight cancer. Pour a dressing that combines these two winners on top of a salad of greens and how can you go wrong? The fresh herbs are what really make this dressing, so try to use fresh, not dried.

½ cup extra-virgin olive oil	1 large clove garlic, minced
3 tablespoons balsamic vinegar	1 tablespoon chopped fresh rosemary
¼ cup roasted red peppers, chopped (jarred or fresh)	1 tablespoon chopped fresh flat-leaf parsley
1 teaspoon honey	Salt and pepper
¼ cup chopped fresh basil, chopped	

Combine all ingredients in a blender and blend until smooth.

Sun-Dried Tomato Salad Dressing

Sun-dried tomatoes are high in Vitamins A and C and a good source of potassium. Tomatoes are rich in lycopene, which may help protect against certain types of cancer, including colorectal, prostate, breast, endometrial, lung, and pancreatic. The health benefits notwithstanding, this savory dressing is fit for the most discerning gourmet palate!

3 sun-dried tomato halves
in olive oil, drained
3 tablespoons balsamic vinegar
1 clove garlic, minced

1 teaspoon capers
⅓ cup extra-virgin olive oil
1 tablespoon chopped,
fresh basil leaves

Place all ingredients in a blender and blend until smooth.

Tapenade and Tomato Salad Dressing

Black olives and tomatoes are both powerhouses of nutrients. This is an easy recipe and a nice way to use up left over tapenade from last night's get together!

¼ cup *Black Olive Tapenade*
¼ cup balsamic vinegar
⅓ cup extra-virgin olive oil

1 medium tomato, seeded and diced
1 clove garlic, minced
1 tablespoon minced fresh basil

Whisk together all ingredients until blended.

Strawberry Basil Vinaigrette

Strawberries could well be one of the healthiest fruits we can eat. Loaded with antioxidants, they are usually available year-round and are also very versatile.

¼ cup extra-virgin olive oil
2 tablespoons balsamic vinegar
8 medium strawberries
Juice of 1 small orange

1 teaspoon honey
2 tablespoons fresh basil
½ teaspoon Dijon mustard
Salt and pepper

Combine all ingredients except olive oil in a blender and blend until smooth. On low speed, gradually add olive oil until fully emulsified.

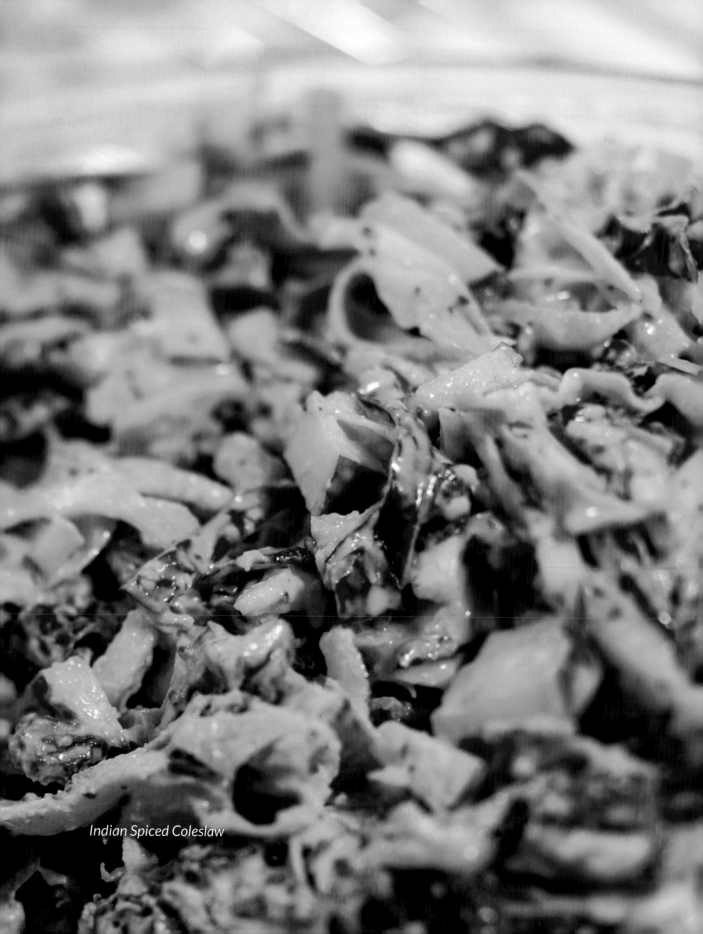

Indian Spiced Coleslaw

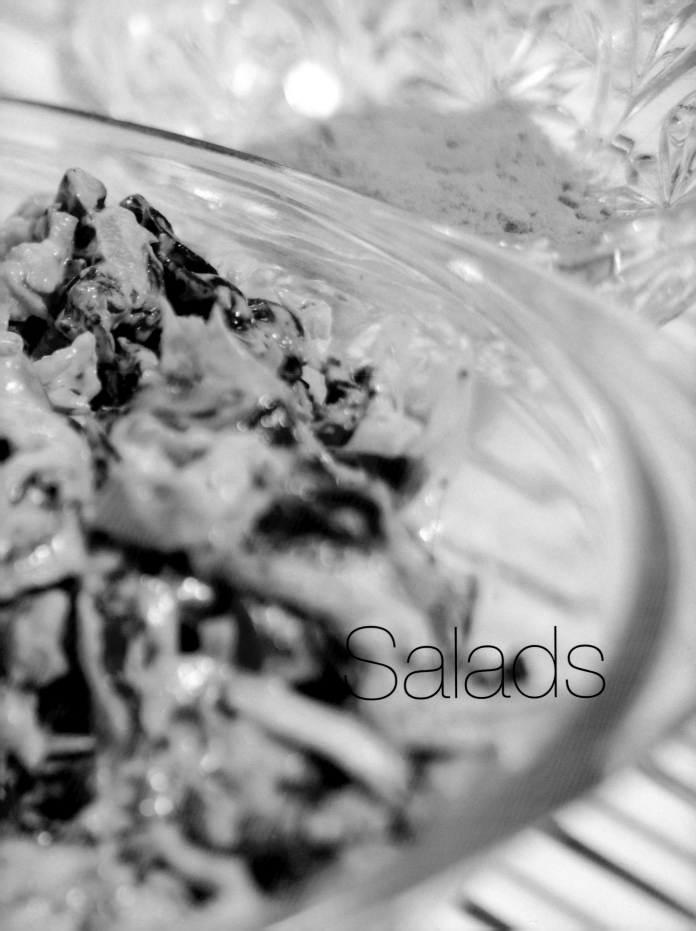

Salads

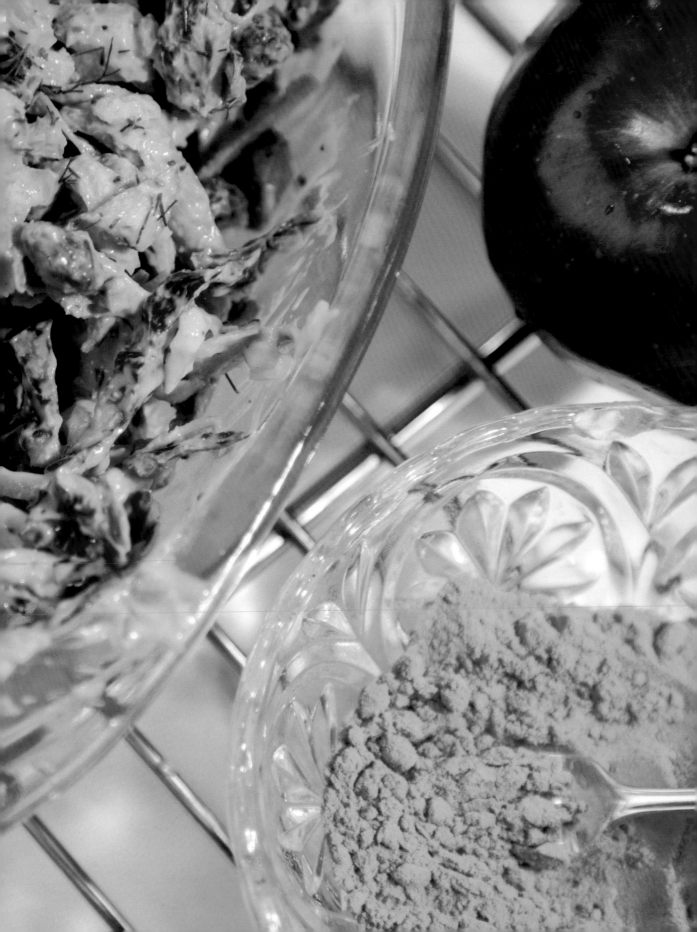

We assume we're eating healthfully when we're chomping down on a salad, but a lot of the time there's enough fat in the salad dressing to sink a ship and can turn salads into a nutritional nightmare!

I eat a salad almost every day for lunch, but I make sure to prepare it so that it's healthy. At the start of the week, I dice and chop my vegetables and then refrigerate them so they're ready to include in my lunchtime salads, whether I'm eating at home or packing my lunch to go. Admittedly, this takes a little prep, but once you get in the swing of things it's a cinch to do.

Salads can be delicious comfort food and a big time cancer preventer, but we have to change our way of thinking about them and what goes into them. With the right ingredients, they're anything but boring and make a very satisfying meal. First of all, ditch the iceberg lettuce—it's mostly water. Instead, use hearty greens like kale, Swiss chard, and raw spinach. Mix it up with some darker leaf lettuces like baby greens or radicchio. Grill your vegetables first, then chill them—or not. The possibilities of interesting, good-tasting salads are endless. I've included some of my favorites here.

Arugula, Mushrooms, and Marinated Tomatoes

Arugula's dark green leaves are members of the cruciferous family, which makes these hearty greens closely related to broccoli, bokchoy, and Brussels sprouts. The cruciferous family of vegetables includes some of the most potent anti-cancer foods around. Arugula has a peppery, mustardy flavor, which makes for an interesting, great tasting salad.

2 cups tomatoes, chopped
¼ cup fresh basil, chopped
3 cloves garlic, minced
2 cups fresh arugula

1 cup fresh mushrooms, sliced
4 tablespoons extra-virgin olive oil
2 tablespoons balsamic vinegar
Salt and pepper

Combine tomatoes, basil, olive oil, balsamic vinegar, and salt and pepper. Allow to marinate in the refrigerator for at least 8 hours. Combine tomatoes with arugula and mushrooms. Mix well and serve cold.

Serves 2

Asparagus and Tomato Salad

Asparagus is not only a wonderful seasonal treat, it has a whopping number of vitamins and nutrients. It is high in glutathione, a nutrient that has been proven in laboratories to help fight certain cancers, and Vitamins A and C. This is a great accompaniment to a summer picnic or barbecue.

1 pound asparagus, trimmed and washed
¼ cup extra-virgin olive oil
4 cloves garlic, minced
2 cups tomatoes, chopped

¼ cup chopped fresh basil
¼ cup extra-virgin olive oil
2 tablespoons balsamic vinegar
Salt and pepper

Coat asparagus with 2 tablespoons extra-virgin olive oil, garlic, and salt and pepper. Cook on a medium hot grill or in an oven heated to 400 degrees F. turning often until brown, tender, and completely roasted. Remove from grill or oven and allow to thoroughly cool. Chop into 1 inch pieces. Set aside.

Combine tomatoes, basil, remaining olive oil, balsamic vinegar, salt and pepper. Mix well. Add chopped asparagus to tomato mixture. Salt and pepper to taste. Allow to marinate in the refrigerator for at least 8 hours. Serve cold by itself or over a salad made with dark green leafy vegetables such as arugula or spinach.

Serves 2

Avocado and Tomato Salad Topping

This salad is really just guacamole with marinated tomatoes, but when you mix the two together you get an especially full-flavored combination. It's great to top a salad with or to use as a dip. Either way you choose to use it, it's worthwhile to remember that the avocado is high in the carotenoids lutein and zeaxanthin, both of which are powerful antioxidants and have cancer-fighting properties. The onion, tomato, and cilantro also all have cancer-fighting properties.

2 cups tomatoes, chopped
1 small onion, minced
3 cloves garlic, minced
2 tablespoons extra-virgin olive oil
¼ cup balsamic vinegar

2 ripe avocados
Juice from 1 lime
¼ cup chopped fresh cilantro
Salt and pepper

Place tomatoes, onion, garlic, olive oil, and balsamic vinegar in a bowl and mix well. Salt and pepper to taste. Place in the refrigerator and allow to marinate for at least 4 hours. Once marinated, remove from refrigerator and drain.

Cut the avocados in half. Scoop out the pulp of the avocado and place in a bowl. Mash well. Add the lime juice and cilantro. Mix in the tomato mixture and stir well. Salt and pepper to taste. Serve cold.

Serves 2-3

Brown Rice Curry Salad

This is an interesting, crunchy salad that has the extra perk of curry. Curry, walnuts, onions, and whole grains have all been shown to have properties that help fight cancer.

1 cup *Yogurt Cheese*
1 tablespoon curry powder
2 cups cooked brown rice
1 green onion, diced
1 apple, cored and diced
1 large stalk celery, diced

¼ cup dried cranberries
¼ cup raisins
¼ cup walnuts, chopped and toasted
1 tablespoon raw brown sugar
2 tablespoons canola oil
Salt and pepper

In a small bowl, mix together the *Yogurt Cheese* and curry powder. In a large bowl, combine all other ingredients and mix well. Toss together with the yogurt mixture. Combine well. Serve cold.

Serves 3-4

Barley and Vegetable Salad

This little lesser-used grain of barley is high in fiber and can help prevent several diseases—everything from gall bladder disease to diabetes to heart problems. Barley contains antioxidants and phytochemicals too, both of which help prevent cancer. This is a very versatile salad. You can pretty much use whatever vegetables, cooked or raw, that might be sitting in your refrigerator.

1 small onion, chopped
1 tablespoon olive oil
1 cup barley, uncooked
3 cups vegetable broth or low-fat chicken broth
1 small onion, chopped
1 (16 ounce) can garbanzo beans (chickpeas), rinsed and drained
1 large tomato, chopped
1 red pepper, seeded and chopped

1 green pepper, seeded and chopped
1 small cucumber, chopped
1 large garlic clove, minced
¼ cup chopped fresh flat-leaf parsley
¼ cup chopped fresh cilantro
½ cup chopped fresh mint
½ cup diced celery
Juice of 1 lime
Salt and pepper

In a large skillet, over medium heat, brown onion in oil until soft. Add barley, stirring often, and cook until barley is slightly brown. Add broth and bring to a boil. Reduce heat to a simmer, cover skillet, and cook until barley is tender, about 45 minutes.

When barley is done to your liking (I like mine al dente), remove from heat and let stand for 10 minutes. Place in the refrigerator until cold.

When barley is chilled, mix it together in a large bowl with all other ingredients. Toss well, but gently, and place back in the refrigerator for at least 2 hours to chill again and for the flavors to meld. Salt and pepper to taste.

Serve with *Creamy Cilantro Salad Dressing* or *Minced Herb Salad Dressing*.

Serves 3-4

Beet Salad

Most of us think of beets as red vegetables, but they also come in white and yellow (golden). I've included some golden beets in this recipe, but if you can't find them, you can use all red beets instead. Red beets may prove to be a powerful cancer-fighting food. The pigment that gives beets their rich red color is betacyanin, and it's been shown in several studies to be an effective cancer fighter.

2 large red beets	1 teaspoon Dijon mustard
2 large golden beets	¼ cup walnuts, chopped
¼ cup chopped fresh basil	3 cups arugula
3 tablespoons extra-virgin olive oil	Salt and pepper
3 tablespoons balsamic vinegar	

Preheat the oven to 425 degrees F. Trim the tops and roots from the beets and wash the vegetables very well. Separate the golden beets from the red beets. Cut two large pieces of aluminum foil (large enough to fold over and seal beets in). Place the red beets in the center of one piece of foil and the golden beets in the center of the other piece of foil. Fold each piece of foil over and seal each packet so beets are tightly enclosed in the foil packets. Place the beet packets on a cookie sheet, and bake in the preheated oven until the beets are soft, about 1 hour.

Test if they are cooked by poking a beet, through the foil, with the top of a sharp knife. If the knife glides in smoothly, the beets are done. Remove from the oven and allow the beets to cool while still in foil. When the beets are cool enough to handle, open the foil packets carefully. Run the beets under cold water while rubbing them, and the skin will peel off easily. Still keeping the beets separate, slice the beets and place the red beets in a small bowl and the golden beets in another small bowl.

In another large bowl, whisk together the olive oil, balsamic vinegar, and mustard. Add the beets, basil, and walnuts and toss gently. Salt and pepper to taste. Serve on a bed of arugula.

Serves 3-4

Carrot and Raisin Salad

Results from studies in laboratories have shown that eating carrots helps reduce the risk of getting cancer. Your mother always told you they were good for you, didn't she? There is a natural pesticide in carrots called falcarinol that protects carrots from fungal diseases. Carrots are virtually the only way we can obtain this chemical through our human diet and this compound, when the carrots are raw, has been shown to help curb cancer.

4 cups carrots, shredded
1 cup pineapple (fresh or canned) diced
1 large apple, diced
1 cup raisins
¼ cup walnuts, chopped
¼ cup celery, chopped

1 cup *Yogurt Cheese* (drained in the refrigerator for 24 hours)
3 tablespoons light mayonnaise
1 tablespoon raw brown sugar
Salt and pepper

In a large bowl, mix all of the ingredients well. Serve chilled. This salad is even better if it is allowed to sit in the refrigerator overnight, so the flavors have an opportunity to meld together.

Serves 3-4

Cole Slaw

This is a more traditional slaw than the Indian spiced slaw, but it's also a heavy hitter anti-cancer wise. It contains several cancer-fighting foods.

Slaw

4 cups red cabbage, shredded
4 cups green cabbage, shredded
1 medium red onion, sliced very thin
2 carrots, shredded
1 cup raisins
2 apples, diced
Salt and pepper

Sauce

3 cups *Yogurt Cheese* (drained in the refrigerator for 24 hours)
3 tablespoons canola oil or light olive oil
¼ cup raw brown sugar
½ cup apple cider vinegar
1 tablespoon celery seeds
1 tablespoon mustard seeds
2 cloves garlic, minced

In a large bowl, mix all of the slaw ingredients well. In a smaller bowl, whisk together all of the sauce ingredients until blended. Add the sauce to the slaw ingredients and mix well. Salt and pepper to taste. Serve chilled. This is even better if it sits in the refrigerator overnight, so the flavors have an opportunity to meld together.

Serves 4-6

Citrus Salad with Ginger Dressing

Citrus fruits are loaded with Vitamin C and fiber. A study in Japan found citrus consumption to be associated with reduced incidences of most cancers. This is a pretty salad, great for summertime or to help perk you up out of wintertime doldrums.

2 tangerines
1 navel orange
1 pink grapefruit
1 cup fresh pineapple, chopped
1 apple, cut in chunks
2 chives, chopped finely
¼ cup walnuts, chopped

½ cup *Yogurt Cheese*
1 teaspoon grated fresh ginger root
Juice of one orange
Zest of one orange
1 tablespoon tahini
1 tablespoon honey
Salt and pepper

Peel the tangerines, orange, and grapefruit, making sure to remove as much of the white pith as possible. Slice into bite-size chunks. Place in a bowl along with pineapple, apple, chives, and walnuts and toss well. In a small bowl, combine *Yogurt Cheese*, ginger root, orange juice, zest, tahini, and honey to make ginger dressing. Whisk until blended. Salt and pepper to taste. Pour over fruit and mix well. Serve chilled.

Serves 3-4

Chopped Salad

Most chopped salads are made with iceberg lettuce, which is mostly water. This chopped salad is made with kale and arugula, members of the cruciferous family that have shown to help prevent some cancers. I love the texture of a chopped salad. This is a mix-and-match salad. Choose the vegetables you desire. Just make sure to chop all of them finely. Top with your favorite dressing and enjoy!

1 cup kale, chopped finely
1 cup spinach, chopped finely
1 cup arugula, chopped finely
½ pound button mushrooms, chopped finely
2 large tomatoes, seeded, chopped finely
1 large carrot, chopped finely
1 large celery stalk, chopped finely

½ cup black olives, chopped finely
1 red onion, chopped finely
1 (15½ ounce) can garbanzo beans (chickpeas), drained
¼ cup chopped fresh basil
1 tablespoon chopped fresh oregano

Place all ingredients in a large bowl and combine well. Toss with salad dressing and serve cold.

Serves 3-4

Egg White Egg Salad

Every now and then I just get a yen for an old-fashioned egg salad sandwich. Although I no longer eat the fat that normally comes with the old-fashioned version, I can still satisfy the craving. You'll never miss the yolks, as there's plenty of flavor here!

8 large eggs
¼ cup celery, chopped
¼ cup onions, chopped
¼ cup red bell pepper, chopped
¼ cup tomatoes, chopped

1 small carrot, grated
1 tablespoon nonfat mayonnaise dressing
3 tablespoons *Yogurt Cheese*
1 teaspoon Dijon mustard
Salt and pepper

Place eggs in a saucepan. Cover with enough cold water to cover 1 inch above the eggs. Heat rapidly to boiling. Reduce heat and simmer for 10 minutes. Remove from heat and rinse the eggs in cold water to stop further cooking. Tap egg to crack shell, and peel off eggshell.

Discard the yolks, reserving the whites. Chop the whites. Combine the chopped egg whites with all other ingredients, and mix well. Salt and pepper to taste. Refrigerate until chilled. Serve on *Plain Ol' Whole Wheat Bread* or inside *Whole Wheat Pita* for a sandwich.

Serves 3-4

Fennel Salad

Fennel is a much under-used vegetable in the United States, but it shouldn't be. It has a delicious, mild licorice flavor and is high in antioxidants. Fennel is also high in fiber and in Vitamin C and contains the phytonutrient compound anethole. In studies, anethole has been shown to reduce inflammation and to help prevent the occurrence of cancer. This makes for a scrumptious salad treat.

2 fennel bulbs, cut in ¼ inch strips
3 oranges, peeled and cut in pieces
¼ cup raisins
1 red onion, thinly sliced

2 tablespoons olive oil
2 tablespoons red wine vinegar
1 teaspoon Dijon mustard
Salt and pepper

Combine the fennel, oranges, raisins, and onion in a large bowl. In a smaller bowl, whisk together the oil, vinegar, mustard, and salt and pepper to create a vinaigrette. Pour the vinaigrette over the fennel mixture and toss to combine. Serve cold.

Serves 2-3

Indian Spiced Cole Slaw

This is a quadruple hitter, as it has four cancer fighters in it: cabbage, garlic, onions, and turmeric! It also has omega-3s from the oil. Besides all of that, it tastes pretty darn good. Its interesting flavors make for a great side dish or a first course salad.

Slaw	Sauce
2 cups red cabbage, shredded	1 cup *Yogurt Cheese* (drained in the refrigerator for 24 hours)
2 cups green cabbage, shredded	2 tablespoons canola oil or light olive oil
1 small fennel bulb, shredded	2 cloves garlic, crushed
1 small red onion, thinly sliced	1 tablespoon raw brown sugar
1 carrot, shredded	Juice of 1 lemon
½ cup raisins	1 teaspoon cumin
1 large apple, diced	1 tablespoon turmeric
Salt and pepper	2 tablespoons tahini sauce
	1 tablespoon celery seed

In a large bowl, mix all of the slaw ingredients well. In a small bowl, whisk together all of the sauce ingredients until blended. Add the sauce to the slaw ingredients and mix well. Salt and pepper to taste.

Serve chilled. This is even better if it sits in the refrigerator overnight so the flavors get a chance to meld together. It lasts a week in the refrigerator and still tastes fresh.

Serves 4-6

Note: For a real gourmet treat, mix this cole slaw 50/50 with a garden salad and dress with olive oil and vinegar. Makes a terrific lunchtime salad!

Potato Salad

Potatoes aren't really bad for you. They have gotten a bad reputation because of the unhealthy ways they are sometimes prepared along with the unhealthy toppings that are usually piled on. White potatoes actually contain vitamins, minerals, and phytochemicals. Sweet potatoes contain beta-carotene and Vitamin C and are an antioxidant rich food. So go ahead and enjoy this healthier version of an old favorite at your next barbecue or picnic.

3 large unpeeled Idaho potatoes
1 large peeled sweet potato,
cut in 1 inch cubes
1 large onion, diced
2 stalks celery, diced
3 large cloves garlic, minced
1 red pepper, seeded and diced
1 green pepper, seeded and diced

1 cup *Yogurt Cheese* (drained in the refrigerator for 24 hours)
¼ cup light mayonnaise
¼ cup chopped flat-leaf parsley
2 tablespoons chopped fresh dill
2 tablespoons olive oil
1 small jalapeño pepper, seeded and chopped very finely (optional)
Salt and pepper

Prick Idaho potatoes with a fork and cook in the microwave until soft. Remove and allow to cool until you can handle them easily. Once cool enough to touch, cut into 1 inch cubes.

Cook the sweet potato in the microwave until soft. Set aside.

In a large skillet, combine the olive oil, garlic, and the onions. Cook over medium heat, stirring often, until onions begin to caramelize, about 20 minutes. Remove from heat and allow to cool.

In a large bowl, combine the potatoes and onions along with all of the other ingredients. Mix well. Salt and pepper to taste. Serve chilled.

Serves 4-6

Kale, Tomato, and Avocado Salad

This is a really lovely salad. The flavors meld together wonderfully in a flavorful and healthy dish.

2 cups tomatoes, diced
2 cloves garlic, crushed
2 tablespoons fresh chopped basil
2 tablespoons olive oil

2 tablespoons balsamic vinegar
1 large bunch kale, cleaned and cut up
1 ripe avocado, diced
Salt and pepper

Combine tomatoes, garlic, and basil. Add the olive oil and balsamic vinegar. Mix well. Refrigerate for a minimum of two hours, allowing the tomatoes time to marinate.

After marinating tomatoes, add them to the kale along with avocado. Mix well. Salt and pepper to taste.

Serves 2

Marinated Tomatoes

Tomatoes contain lycopene, which is a free radical-fighting antioxidant. This little side dish also contains garlic and olive oil, both of which are cancer-fighting foods. Besides being healthy for you, these tomatoes are so simple to prepare, and they really perk up any meal with their full, savory flavor. I serve this as a side, over a little lettuce or in a mixed salad. So easy, so good, and so good for you.

1 pound tomatoes, chopped (I like to vary my types to achieve a variety of tastes. I use a mix of cherry, plum, yellow, and black tomatoes. Mix it up with whatever tomatoes are in season and don't be afraid to try something new.)

1 large clove garlic, crushed
¼ cup chopped fresh basil
¼ cup chopped fresh cilantro
2 tablespoons balsamic vinegar
2 tablespoons extra-virgin olive oil
Salt and pepper

Mix all ingredients together and let the mixture sit in the refrigerator for an hour or so before serving, as the flavors need a little time to meld together. Stir again before serving.

Salt and pepper to taste.

Serves 2-3

Roasted Broccoli Salad

Broccoli is rich in Vitamin C, carotenoids, fiber, calcium, and folate. It's also a great source of the phytochemicals that are being studied for their anti-cancer properties. This salad is healthy, delicious, and a company favorite.

4 cups broccoli florets, cooked to al dente texture, drained and cooled
¼ cup olive oil
3 cloves garlic, minced
3 tablespoons roasted, unsalted sunflower seeds

1 red onion, diced
1 celery stalk, diced
1 cup canned garbanzo beans (chickpeas), rinsed and drained
3 tablespoons raisins
Salt and pepper

Preheat oven to 400 degrees F. In a large bowl, coat the broccoli florets well with olive oil and minced garlic. Spread the florets out on a cookie sheet or in a roasting pan and place in the oven to roast, turning occasionally until cooked to a tender crisp texture (al dente). Remove from oven and allow to cool. Once cool, place florets in a large bowl and mix with all remaining ingredients. Toss gently but well to combine all ingredients. Salt and pepper to taste. Top with *Creamy Cilantro Dressing* and serve cold.

Serves 4

Spinach, Mushroom, and Grilled Onion Salad

This is a classic spinach salad (without the bacon!) with a twist. Grilling the onions first and serving them warm atop the salad gives another whole layer of flavor to the dish. Spinach is loaded with vitamins, minerals, and phytonutrients and has been shown to help prevent several kinds of cancer.

1 large red onion, sliced
1 tablespoon olive oil
12 ounces pre-washed baby spinach

8 ounces white mushrooms, sliced
¼ cup dried cherries, no sugar added
¼ cup walnuts, chopped and toasted

In a small skillet, sauté the onions in the olive oil over a low heat. Cook until the onions begin to caramelize (about 20 minutes). Remove from stove. While the onions are cooking, in a large bowl, mix together the spinach, mushrooms, cherries, and walnuts. Toss in the caramelized onions and dress with *Honey Mustard Dressing* or *Poppy Seed Dressing*. Serve immediately while onions are still warm.

Serves 3-4

Roasted Corn Salad

Corn has been around for literally hundreds of years, and there is a good reason for its longevity. It's low in saturated fat and cholesterol and a good source of fiber. Corn comes in several varieties, yellow, white, blue, purple, and red. Roasting corn on the grill is an irresistible summertime treat. Unlike a piece of meat, you can grill your veggies to your heart's content without any worries of carcinogens forming.

6 large ears corn on the cob, husked
3 cloves garlic, minced
2 tablespoons chopped fresh cilantro
2 tablespoons chopped fresh flat-leaf parsley
1 red pepper, chopped
1 green pepper, chopped
1 small cucumber, peeled, seeded, and chopped

3 green onions, chopped
1 small red onion, chopped
1 lemon, juice and zest
1 lime, juice and zest
1 celery stalk, chopped finely
½ cup extra-virgin olive oil
¼ cup balsamic vinegar
Olive oil spray
Salt and pepper

Preheat grill to high. Spray the cobs with olive oil spray until well coated.

Place on the preheated grill for 5 minutes and then reduce the heat to medium. Continue to roast the cobs, turning often until the corn is nicely brown and tender.

Remove from grill and allow to cool. Once cool, cut the roasted corn off of the cob and discard the cobs. Put the corn into a large bowl. Add all of the remaining ingredients. Toss well until all of the vegetables are well coated. Salt and pepper to taste. Serve cold.

Serves 4-6

Roasted Vegetable Salad

This is a versatile salad that can be made with almost any vegetable combination, but I like root vegetables. Some research has shown that eating root vegetables might decrease the risk of kidney cancer. Root vegetables are easy to cook, economical, and have a long shelf life in the refrigerator. This salad makes for a hearty plate on a winter's night.

2 large carrots, peeled, cut in slices
1 large onion, cut in 1 inch chunks
6 red potatoes, quartered
1 leak, trimmed, rinsed, and chopped
½ cup olive oil
2 medium beets, peeled,
cut in ½ inch chunks

2 fennel bulbs, tops removed, and cut in ½ inch chunks
4 cloves garlic, minced
¼ cup balsamic vinegar
¼ cup chopped fresh flat-leaf parsley
¼ cup chopped fresh chives
Olive oil spray
Salt and pepper

Preheat the oven to 350 degrees F.

In a large mixing bowl, combine carrots, onion, potatoes, leak, fennel, and garlic and toss with ¼ cup of the olive oil. Spread the vegetables on the bottom of a roasting pan or large cookie sheet and place in the oven. Roast for about 1 hour, turning the vegetables with a spatula occasionally.

Place the beets on a smaller cookie sheet. Spray well with olive oil and put in the oven on another rack (the beets need to be cooked separately, so that the beet color doesn't spread). Roast for about 1 hour also, turning the beets with a spatula occasionally.

When the vegetables are tender, remove from the oven and place in a large bowl (do not add the beets). Allow to cool for about 20 minutes. Add the remaining olive oil along with the balsamic vinegar, parsley, and chives and toss well. Salt and pepper to taste. Gently fold in the beets and refrigerate for at least 8 hours to thoroughly chill.

Serve over a bed of hearty greens.

Serves 6

Salmon Salad

This is a favorite of mine in the summertime. You can put whatever ingredients you like into the salad, but I like to keep this dish pretty simple so the flavors of the salmon and the salad dressing stand out.

Salmon is an excellent source of omega-3 fatty acids, and research has shown that omega-3s reduce inflammation and might lower the risk of cancer. Cruciferous vegetables also have anti-cancer properties, and arugula is considered a cruciferous vegetable.

4 (4 ounce) wild salmon fillets
½ teaspoon granulated garlic
Salt and pepper
3 cups arugula
2 cups baby greens
2 medium tomatoes, diced

½ cucumber, sliced thinly
6 fresh basil leaves, sliced thinly
½ cup black olives, pitted
Honey Mustard Salad Dressing
Olive oil spray

Cooking fish on a high heat, just like meats, can be carcinogenic, so the trick to cooking the fish is to do it in foil over a low heat.

Preheat grill on a low heat or oven to 300 degrees F.

Wash the fish fillets well and spray them with olive oil spray. Salt and pepper the fish and sprinkle on the granulated garlic. Wrap the fish in foil (individually or grouped together) and place on the grill or in the oven. Cook until done, about 10-15 minutes depending on the size of the fillet.

While fish is cooking, in a large bowl, toss together arugula, baby greens, tomatoes, cucumbers, basil, and olives. Toss well with *Honey Mustard Dressing*. Salt and pepper to taste. Divide salads equally onto 4 large plates.

When fish is done, remove from foil and set atop individual salads.

Serve with crusty *Garlic Bread*.

Serves 4

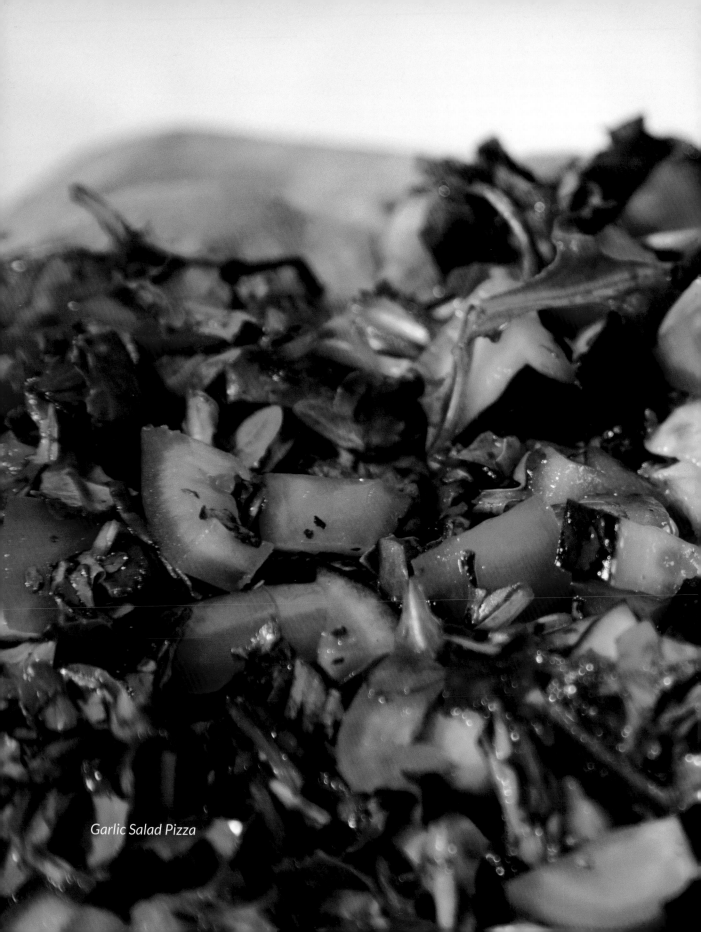

Garlic Salad Pizza

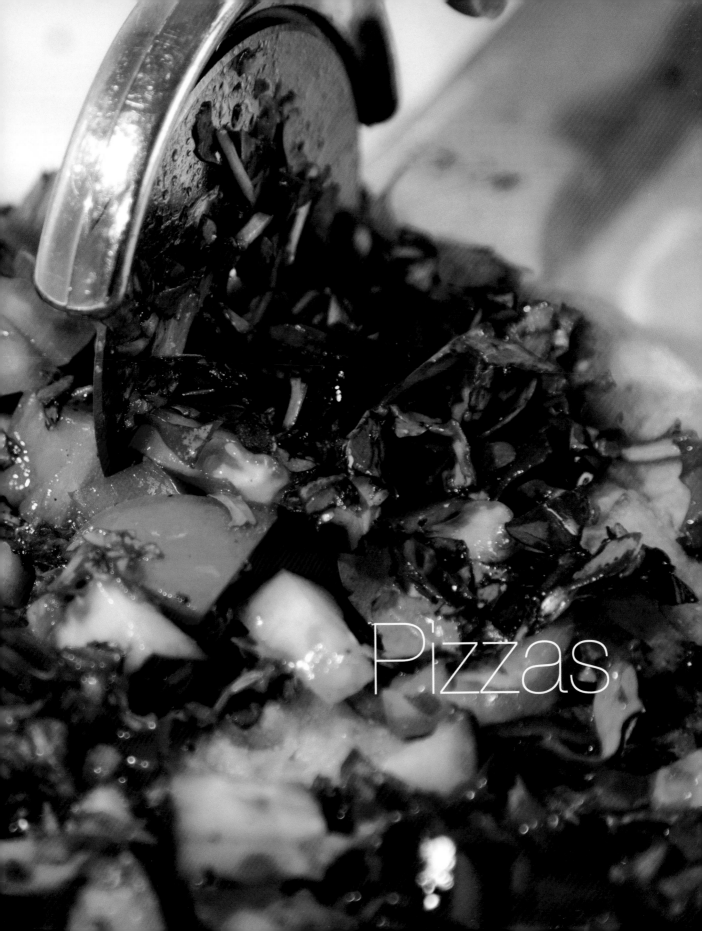

Pizzas

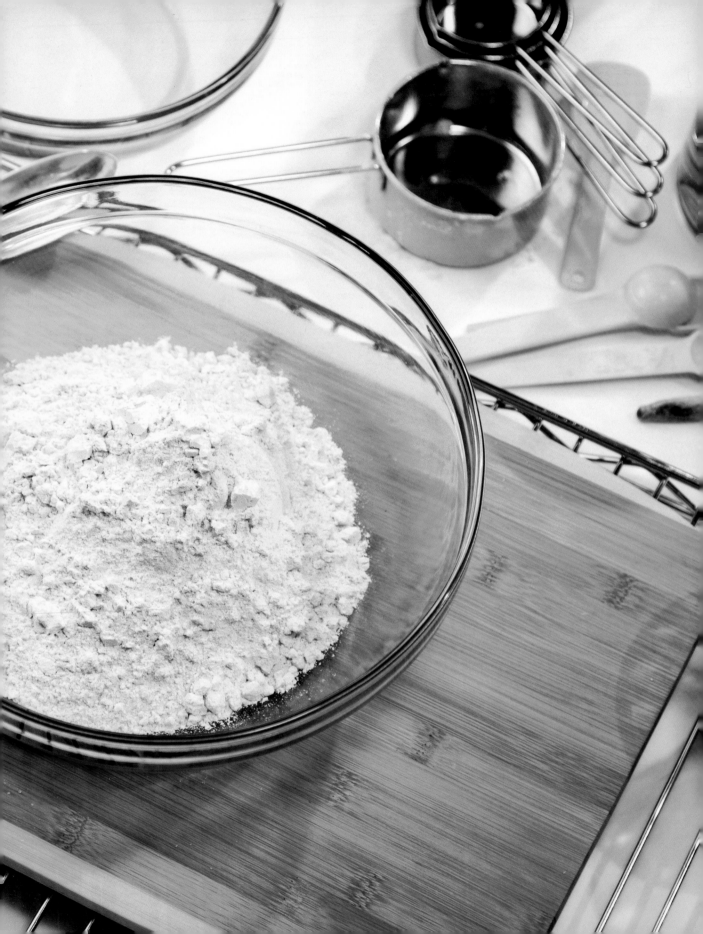

I love pizzas. They are so versatile, and you are only limited by your imagination! I have included a recipe for a whole wheat pizza dough that is easy to make and freezes well. I like to keep a couple of dough balls in the freezer ready to thaw for a quick and easy dinner. Or you can use store bought pizza dough if you can find ones made with healthful ingredients. It might not be easy to do, as most commercial pizza doughs are made with white flour, sugar, and hydrogenated oils, and you want to stay away from those. You're much better off making a couple of batches of your own and freezing them for later use.

Although I make my own pizza sauce, you can cheat if you're in a hurry and use a store-bought sauce. Any strictly veggie, low-fat, pizza or spaghetti sauce will work. If you have the time though, homemade is so much better, and only takes about 10-15 minutes to prepare. I've included my go-to recipe.

I love to make pizzas on the grill. If you have one, you'll see it keeps the mess in the kitchen to a minimum. It's a really fun way to cook, and you get to use your grill without worrying about carcinogens! If you don't have a grill, you can still make these in the oven. I use a pizza paddle to take my pizzas easily in and out of the oven, but if you don't have a pizza paddle, you can place the dough on a cooling rack and place the cooling rack directly into the oven or grill.

I have included some of my favorite recipes, but the possibilities are endless. Think outside of pepperoni and cheese and pizzas can be a healthy, wonderful addition to your diet. This is a great way to get your veggies!

Whole Wheat Pizza Crust

2 packages active dry yeast
¾ cup water (110-115 F.)
3½ cups white whole wheat flour
2 teaspoons raw brown sugar
¾ cup nonfat or soy milk (110-115 F.)

1 teaspoon salt
1 tablespoon olive oil
Whole wheat flour for dusting
Cornmeal for rolling out 12 inch circle
Olive oil spray

Dissolve yeast in a small bowl with water. Allow to sit for 10 minutes.

Place flour, raw brown sugar, and salt in a bowl and mix well (you can use a mixer with a dough hook or you can do it the old fashioned way, by hand). Slowly add milk, yeast, and oil while mixing, until dough comes together in a ball.

Sprinkle flour on table top and place dough on work surface. Knead until dough is smooth, about five minutes. Spray a large bowl with olive oil spray. Place dough in bowl, cover with plastic wrap, and allow to sit in a warm place until dough doubles in size, about one hour. Punch dough down, and allow to rise again, about 30 minutes.

Split dough into four balls. Each will make a 12 inch pizza. Sprinkle your work space with the cornmeal. Roll the dough out and stretch into a 12 inch circle. If you own a pizza paddle, sprinkle the paddle with cornmeal and transfer the rolled out dough onto it or place pizza dough on a cooling rack. You're ready to start loading it up with the good stuff!

Makes four (12 inch) crusts

Pizza Sauce

Remember, tomatoes, garlic, and basil have all been shown to probably prevent certain cancers.

6 medium tomatoes, diced
1 large clove garlic, minced
¼ cup chopped fresh basil
½ teaspoon dried oregano

1 cup tomato sauce
1 teaspoon raw brown sugar
Salt and pepper
Olive oil spray

Spray a skillet with olive oil spray. Add tomatoes and garlic. Simmer on low heat until the water evaporates from the tomatoes. Add remaining ingredients and simmer about 5 minutes. Set aside.

Covers four (12 inch) pizzas

Garlic Salad Pizza

Who would think of putting salad on your pizza? I would! This pizza utilizes a basic mixed salad recipe, but feel free to be creative and modify it to match your taste.

1 *Whole Wheat Pizza Crust*
3 tablespoons olive oil
3 cloves garlic, chopped
1 medium onion, chopped
2 tablespoons low-fat grated Parmesan cheese
¼ cup shredded cheese (part-skim mozzarella, veggie, or soy)
Cornmeal for dusting

1 cup arugula greens
1 cup mixed salad greens
2 tomatoes, chopped
½ cucumber, sliced thinly
¼ cup chopped fresh basil
3 tablespoons olive oil
3 tablespoons balsamic vinegar
Salt and pepper

Preheat oven to 400 degrees F. Heat 1 tablespoon olive oil and onion in a small skillet over a medium heat. Cook until onion is translucent. Stir in the garlic and set aside to cool.

Sprinkle a pizza paddle with a little cornmeal. Place the rolled out pizza dough onto the paddle or place pizza dough onto a cooling rack that is at least as large as the rolled out dough. Using the paddle, slide the dough directly onto the oven rack in the center of preheated oven, or place the cooling rack in the center of preheated oven. Cook until dough is slightly firm, about 3 minutes. This will allow you to easily slide the pizza off of the paddle or cooling rack once the toppings are on it.

When the dough is slightly firm, carefully remove from oven using the paddle or by removing the cooling rack. Do not turn oven off. Brush dough with remaining olive oil and evenly spread out the garlic/onion mixture over the dough, leaving a ½ inch border. Sprinkle with the two cheeses.

Place pizza back into oven. Continue to cook until the crust is crisp and the cheese melts, about 7-10 more minutes. Check occasionally. While pizza is cooking, in a medium bowl, toss together greens, tomatoes, cucumber, and basil. Dress with olive oil and vinegar. Salt and pepper to taste.

Remove pizza from oven and top with salad. Cut with pizza cutter or large knife.

Serves 2

Grilled Asparagus and Mushroom Pizza

This is an interesting combination and a favorite of mine in the summertime when asparagus is in season. You can use your own imagination here. The veggie choices are practically endless.

1 *Whole Wheat Pizza Crust*
1 bunch asparagus, cut in 1 inch pieces
8 ounces fresh mushrooms, sliced
2 tablespoons olive oil
Salt and pepper

4 large leaves fresh basil, chopped
½ cup *Pizza Sauce*
¾ cup shredded cheese (part-skim mozzarella, veggie, or soy)
Cornmeal for dusting

Preheat oven to 400 degrees F. Combine asparagus and mushrooms in a bowl. Drizzle with olive oil, salt and pepper and mix well to coat vegetables. Place vegetables on the grill in a grill pan and cook until done, or heat in a skillet atop the stove and cook until done. Remove from heat.

Sprinkle a pizza paddle with a little cornmeal. Place the rolled out pizza dough onto the paddle, or place pizza dough onto a cooling rack that is at least as large as the rolled out dough. Using the paddle, slide the dough directly onto the oven rack in the center of preheated oven, or place the cooling rack in the center of preheated oven. Cook until dough is slightly firm, about 3 minutes.

When the dough is slightly firm, carefully remove it from the oven using the paddle or by removing the cooling rack. Spoon Pizza Sauce in center of dough and spread the sauce around, leaving a ½ inch border.

Add vegetables and basil evenly atop pizza. Spread cheese evenly over pizza. Place pizza back into oven. Continue to cook until the crust is crisp and the cheese melts, about 7-10 more minutes. Check occasionally to prevent burning. Place on a large plate, cut with pizza cutter or large knife and enjoy!

Serves 2

Tomato and Basil Pizza

This pizza has just a few very simple ingredients, but it's a winner just the same. It's so tasty in the summer time on the grill when the basil is fresh and varied types of tomatoes are plentiful.

1 *Whole Wheat Pizza Crust*
2 cups cherry tomatoes, cut in half.
4 fresh basil leaves, cleaned and chopped
½ cup *Pizza Sauce*

¾ cup shredded cheese (part-skim mozzarella, veggie, or soy)
Salt and pepper

Preheat oven to 400 degrees F. Sprinkle a pizza paddle with a little cornmeal. Place the rolled out pizza dough onto the paddle or onto a cooling rack that is at least as large as the rolled out dough.

Mexican Pizza

This is a different twist on a classic dish. It has all of the flavors of Mexican food along with the goodness of the beans, onions, and tomatoes.

1 *Whole Wheat Pizza Crust*
1 medium red onion, chopped
¼ cup canned sweet corn, drained
1 tablespoon olive oil
½ (15 ounce) can fat-free refried beans
¼ cup salsa, drained
½ of a (7 ounce) can green chilies
½ cup black olives, chopped

1 cup fresh tomatoes, chopped
¼ cup chopped fresh cilantro
2 tablespoons chopped fresh oregano
¾ cup shredded cheese (part-skim mozzarella, veggie, or soy)
Salt and pepper
Chopped jalapeño to taste (optional)

Preheat oven to 400 degrees F. Sprinkle a pizza paddle with a little cornmeal. Place the rolled out pizza dough onto the paddle or onto a cooling rack that is at least as large as the rolled out dough. Using the paddle, slide the dough directly onto the oven rack in the center of preheated oven, or place the cooling rack in the center of preheated oven. Cook until dough is slightly firm, about 3 minutes.

When the dough is slightly firm, carefully remove from oven using the paddle or by removing the cooling rack. Do not turn oven off. Place refried beans in center of dough and spread beans out over dough, leaving a ½ inch border. Spread salsa on top of the refried beans and green chilies on top of the salsa. Evenly spread cooked onions and tomatoes over the top of other ingredients, then olives over top of the pizza. Sprinkle with cilantro and oregano, then cover with layer of cheese last, still leaving the ½ inch border.

Place pizza back into oven. Continue to cook until the crust is crisp and the cheese melts, about 7-10 more minutes. Check occasionally to prevent burning. Place on a large plate, cut with pizza cutter or large knife, and enjoy!

Serves 2

Using the paddle, slide the dough directly onto the oven rack in the center of preheated oven, or place the cooling rack in the center of preheated oven. Cook until dough is slightly firm, about 3 minutes. When the dough is slightly firm, carefully remove from oven using the pizza paddle or by removing the cooling rack. Do not turn oven off. Spoon *Pizza Sauce* into center of dough and spread the sauce, leaving a ½ inch border. Spread tomatoes and basil evenly over sauce. Salt and pepper to taste. Spread cheese evenly over tomatoes and basil.

Place pizza back into oven. Cook until the crust is crisp and the cheese melts, 7-10 more minutes. Check occasionally to prevent burning. Place on a large plate, slice and enjoy!

Serves 2

Pesto Pizza

Pesto and tomatoes, what could be better? Both have cancer-fighting properties and taste great! Leaving the tomatoes chunky makes for a plump, filling pizza with something delectable to bite into.

1 *Whole Wheat Pizza Crust*
¼ cup *Pesto Sauce*
¾ cup shredded cheese (part-skim mozzarella, veggie, or soy).
4 plum tomatoes, cut in ½ inch chunks

6 ounces of shredded white meat cooked chicken (optional)
Canola oil spray

Sautéed Pepper and Onion Pizza

Back in the days when I ate meat, I used to love an Italian sausage sandwich smothered in sautéed onions and peppers. Italian sausage is no longer in my diet, but the taste of those great peppers doesn't have to be!

1 *Whole Wheat Pizza Crust*
½ green pepper, julienned
½ red pepper, julienned
½ yellow pepper, julienned
1 onion, julienned
4 leaves fresh basil, chopped

1 teaspoon fresh chopped oregano
2 tablespoons olive oil
½ cup *Pizza Sauce*
¾ cup shredded cheese (part-skim mozzarella, veggie, or soy)
Salt and pepper

Preheat oven to 400 degrees F. Place peppers and onions in a bowl. Drizzle with olive oil, salt and pepper. Mix well to coat vegetables. Sauté on a medium heat until al dente. Remove from heat.

Sprinkle a pizza paddle with a little cornmeal. Place the rolled out pizza dough onto the paddle or onto a cooling rack that is at least as large as the rolled out dough. Using the paddle, slide the dough directly onto the oven rack in the center of preheated oven, or place the cooling rack in the center of preheated oven. Cook until dough is slightly firm, about 3 minutes.

When the dough is slightly firm, carefully remove from oven using the paddle or by removing the cooling rack. Do not turn oven off. Spoon *Pizza Sauce* into center of dough and spread around leaving a ½ inch border. Arrange cooked veggies evenly over the sauce, then sprinkle with cheese.

Place pizza back into oven. Cook until the crust is crisp and the cheese melts, about 7-10 more minutes. Check occasionally to prevent burning. Place on a large plate, cut with pizza cutter or large knife, and enjoy!

Serves 2

Preheat oven to 400 degrees F. Sprinkle a pizza paddle with a little cornmeal. Place the rolled out pizza dough onto the paddle or onto a cooling rack that is at least as large as the rolled out dough Using the paddle, slide the dough directly onto the oven rack in the center of preheated oven, or place the cooling rack in the center of preheated oven. Cook until dough is slightly firm, about 3 minutes. When the dough is slightly firm, carefully remove from oven but do not turn oven off. With a large spoon, spread pesto sauce evenly over the pizza leaving ½ inch border. Distribute tomatoes and shredded chicken (if desired) evenly on top of pizza leaving 1/2 inch border. Sprinkle the cheese on top. Return pizza to oven. Cook until the crust is crisp and the cheese melts, about 7-10 more minutes. Check occasionally.

Serves 2

Roasted Vegetable Pizza

I've chosen these vegetables, but use whichever you like.

1 *Whole Wheat Pizza Crust*
5 tablespoons olive oil
2 cups broccoli, cut in 1 inch pieces
2 cups cauliflower, cut in 1 inch pieces
2 carrots, cut in 1 inch pieces
1 onion, cut in 1 inch pieces
1 large tomato, chopped
Salt and pepper

2 large garlic cloves, minced
4 large leaves fresh basil, chopped
1 tablespoon fresh oregano, chopped
¾ cup shredded cheese (part-skim mozzarella, veggie, or soy)
2 tablespoons low-fat grated Parmesan cheese
Cornmeal for dusting

Preheat oven to 400 degrees F. Place broccoli, cauliflower, carrots, and onion in a bowl. Drizzle with olive oil and salt and pepper and mix well to coat vegetables. Place vegetables in a 9" x 13" baking dish, and place in preheated oven. Roast until vegetables are al dente, about 30 minutes. Mix with large spoon occasionally to prevent burning. Remove from oven.

Sprinkle a pizza paddle with a little cornmeal. Place the rolled out pizza dough onto the paddle or onto a cooling rack that is at least as large as the rolled out dough. Using the paddle, slide the dough directly onto the oven rack in the center of preheated oven, or place the cooling rack in the center of preheated oven. Cook until dough is slightly firm, about 3 minutes. This will allow you to easily slide the pizza off of the paddle or cooling rack once the toppings are on it. When the dough is slightly firm, carefully remove from oven using the paddle or by removing the cooling rack. Do not turn oven off.

Mix garlic with 2 tablespoons olive oil and spread the garlic and oil over the pizza dough, leaving a ½ inch border. Sprinkle the oregano and basil evenly over the dough, then add vegetables evenly over herbs and cheese over vegetables. Bake another 7-10 minutes, or until the crust is crisp and the cheese melts. Be sure to check occasionally. Sprinkle with Parmesan cheese, slice, and enjoy!

Serves 2

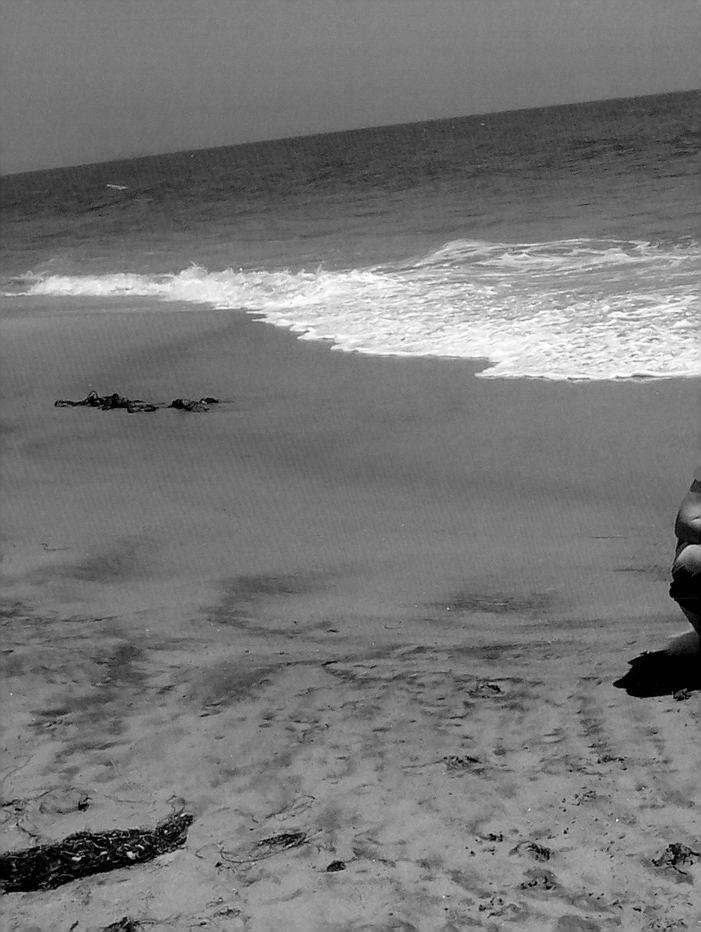

"I am a late-stage cancer survivor who defied the odds and in all probability shouldn't still be here. But I am, and I believe with all of my heart that food is a major reason I survived to write this book."

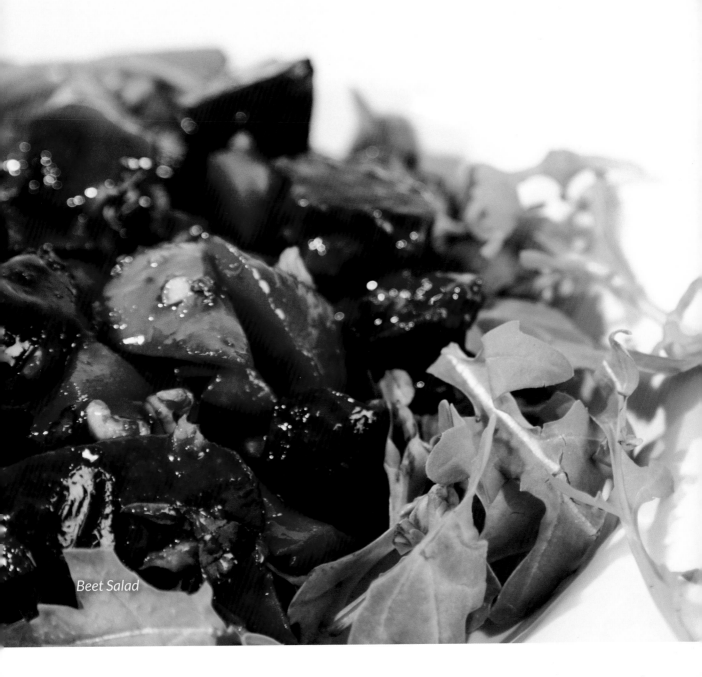

"I always looked forward to chemo days. It meant that I was fighting the cancer. The chemo may have been making me nauseous, but it wasn't making me sick, it was making me healthy."

Beet Salad

My Story

In the summer of 2004, at the age of 52, I was not feeling well. The fact is that I was almost dead and didn't know it. I did know that I was very tired. I remember talking on the phone with my best friend, whom I've known for 40 years, and telling her that I was as tired as I had ever been in my entire life. I had trouble getting through the day and plopped on the couch as soon as I could after getting home from work. I had a steady pain in my back that never went away.

Up until this point, I didn't even have a regular doctor. I had always been healthy and never really needed one. If I got the flu or whatever, I just took myself to a local Urgent Care Center. So I did indeed take myself to the little local clinic thinking I had mononucleosis or the flu. They ran a few tests for the flu, mono, even West Nile virus, and really didn't find anything. I went to a few other doctors and again, the same non-diagnosis.

Meanwhile, I just knew something was wrong. So one day, after a day of increasing discomfort, I went to a local hospital emergency room around 9:00 P.M. and told the emergency doctor everything that I had been through and all of my symptoms. He said, "The symptoms that you're telling me could be anything; I'm running everything." And he did. He ran $12,000 worth of tests in one night—one long night. At 5:30 A.M. the next morning, when I was exhausted from tests and no sleep, he delivered the bad news with a nurse in tow. I knew when I saw the nurse with him that the news was bad. I assumed the doctor was there to deliver the bad news, and the nurse was there to catch me/console me when/if I collapsed. The doctor said it appeared as if I had lymphoma.

I didn't know exactly what lymphoma was or even what a lymph node was, for that matter. I did know I was in trouble and that I had cancer. After a biopsy was done a few days later, my cancer was shown to be gynecological in nature, not lymphoma. It was just present in so many lymph nodes that it appeared to be lymphoma. My new oncologist told me that he would schedule a complete hysterectomy and then biopsy that, and they would then know the origin and type of cancer. He thought it was ovarian cancer that had spread to my lymph nodes. My heart was pounding and terror absolutely filled my soul. *Ovarian cancer that had spread to my lymph nodes*. That did not have a good ring to it.

While I was waiting for my surgery date, my surgeon scheduled me to have a mammogram because he knew the cancer was gynecological; he just was not sure where it originated. It could have been breast cancer. I remember him saying, "If we're lucky, it will be breast cancer." I thought, *If we're lucky it will be breast cancer? Oh my God, how did I get here?* I guess he figured I'd have a better shot of survival if it was breast cancer. So I went in for my mammogram a few days later hoping that I had breast cancer. Bad news—I didn't. The mammogram came back clean.

Two weeks later I had a very successful surgery thanks to the miracle hands of my surgeon. A biopsy was done, and it turned out to be fallopian tube cancer, the rarest of gynecological cancers. There are only approximately 200 new cases in the U.S. a year. At least I now knew what I was dealing with, but it was stage 3c, possibly stage 4.

I remember sitting at my dining room table, absolutely dumbfounded by the news and the statistics because, at the time, I really didn't feel that sick, and saying, "Well, when have I not been in the top percentage of anything I've attempted in life, if I put my mind to it?" There was so little I could control over this disease, but my diet was one big thing I could. So I started my food research.

Although I went the traditional route of surgery and chemotherapy, I supplemented that treatment with diet. I began researching foods that have been tested and shown to help fight or prevent cancer. Seeing that I had been in the restaurant business for years, food and the preparation thereof had become an integral part of my life. Now cancer had, too, so it was only natural that the two of them would combine, and lo and behold, the outcome would be not only be my good health but also this book. I believe that surgery and chemo cured my cancer, but I also believe that changing my diet has kept it from reoccurring. Although the data regarding foods and cancer reoccurrence is mixed and the research is still ongoing, I believe nourishing my body with a primarily plant-based diet has kept me healthy and strong.

Science has produced an overwhelming body of evidence indicating how phytochemicals (nutritive components found in fruits, vegetables, herbs, whole grains, legumes, nuts, and spices) work to prevent cancer. The line between medicine and food is blurring.

Nine years after the dreaded diagnosis in that emergency room at 5:30 A.M., I not only survived, but I'm thriving!

If you are on your own cancer journey, I hope this book will help you through it. If you are not on a cancer journey, I hope this book will deter you from taking the trip in the first place.

Foods to Enjoy

These are foods that I try to include in my daily diet, but again, please check with your doctor or licensed dietician first to make sure they're right for you and any particular nutritional requirements you may have. For instance, there is controversy over consuming soy if you have a history of breast or other hormone-related cancer, controversy over the benefits versus the risks of drinking red wine, and there has also been controversy over the effects of some fats (omega-3s) on some cancers.

So, I would suggest you do some additional research of your own for your daily diet, along with having a consult with your physician. These are foods that have been shown in laboratory tests to help fight cancer, and ones that I try to eat daily. See *Appendix-I* for Study Citations.

Berries are among the fruits highest in antioxidants and are excellent sources of several phytochemicals that seem to help block cancer.

Citrus Fruits contain limonoids, compounds that are usually found in the peels. Preliminary research found limonoids could prevent and halt cancer under laboratory conditions.

Cruciferous Vegetables (including cabbage, broccoli, kale, chard, cauliflower, Brussels sprouts, and collard greens) contain the chemical Indole-3-Carbinol, or I3C for short. Studies have shown that I3C encourages a process called apoptosis, which involves the elimination of damaged cells from your body. Researchers have also found that I3C can help prevent cancer cells from growing.

Dark Chocolate is high in antioxidants. It has to be dark chocolate, not milk chocolate, and at least 70% cacao. If the wrapper says "dark chocolate," but does not list the cacao percentage, it probably is not at least 70% cacao. Before you go jumping for joy about avidly eating this food, remember, moderation is the key. While dark chocolate is good for you, it is also high in fat and calories. It is not recommended to consume more than 1-1½ ounces a day.

Garlic, according to studies, probably protects against stomach cancer and decreases one's chances of developing colon cancer. However, when garlic is chopped and then immediately cooked it loses these possible anti-cancer properties. Always prepare garlic first. If using garlic in a recipe that is going to be crushed, minced, or chopped, allow the cut garlic to sit for at least ten minutes before cooking. Research has shown that letting garlic sit, even for a short amount of time, allows it to retain most of its nutritional value.

Green and White Teas contain two substances, epigallocatechingallate (EGCG) and epigallocatechin (EGC). In laboratories, these have been shown to help prevent cancer.

Herbs and Spices often contain powerful antioxidants. Just one tablespoon of oregano has the same antioxidant activity as a medium sized apple. In recent studies, oregano was found to have even more antioxidants than garlic, long known for its antioxidant properties.

- The fresh herbs with the most antioxidant activity are oregano, sage, peppermint, thyme, lemon balm, and marjoram.
- The dried herbs with the most antioxidant activity are cloves, allspice, cinnamon, rosemary, thyme, marjoram, saffron, oregano, tarragon, and basil.

Omega-3 fatty acids are considered EFAs (essential fatty acids). EFAs are crucial to human health but cannot be manufactured by the body. Therefore, they must be obtained from food. Omega-3 fatty acids can be found in fish and certain plant oils. Walnuts, salmon, soybeans, halibut, shrimp, tofu, winter squash, snapper, scallops, and supplements are good ways to get your omega-3s. If you use supplements, and I do, check to see if your supplements pass the *International Fish Oil Standards Program.*

Onions contain antioxidants—the stronger the onion, the more antioxidants there are. Shallots and Western Yellow contain the highest amount of flavonoids (an antioxidant found in onions). Furthermore, studies have shown that shallots, Northern Red, Western Yellow, and New York Bold onions had the greatest ability to actually slow the growth of cancer.

Red wine is a great source of biologically active phytochemicals, particularly compounds called polyphenols, and these are believed to have anti-cancer properties. However, moderation is the key. I enjoy a 3-4 ounce glass of wine with my dinner, no more. Research has shown that drinking excessive amounts of alcohol is linked to many types of cancer. Nevertheless, there are significant health benefits to drinking red wine in moderation.

Soy foods are rich in phytochemicals, and one group of phytochemicals, isoflavones, may fight cancer in a variety of ways. Isoflavones are only found in soybeans and in soy foods, such as tofu, soy milk, tempeh, and textured soy protein.

Turmeric is a spice commonly used in India. Studies have shown that it contains anti-cancer properties and the ability to reduce cancer growth and decrease metastatic disease. If I don't cook on a given day with this spice, then I fill a gel cap with it and take it as a supplement.

Fruits and Vegetables, in general, are all beneficial and should be included in your diet.. Although the above list contains foods that have been specifically shown to help fight cancer, all vegetables are good for you, and you need to include them in your diet. Mix them up and enjoy them! Remember, only plants contain nutrients called phytochemicals, and research shows that the more phytochemicals you eat, the lower your risk of cancer.

Foods to Avoid

Red Meat (beef, lamb, pork) has been shown in studies to help promote colon cancer, prostate cancer, breast cancer, and lymphoma. In addition, meat that has been char-grilled, blackened, or heavily cooked at high temperatures probably contains carcinogens (agents that cause cancer).

Processed Meat probably promotes several different kinds of colon cancer according to the Second Expert Report, recently published by the American Institute for Cancer Research and the World Cancer Research Fund. Preserving meat by smoking, curing or salting, and/or adding chemical preservatives causes carcinogens to be formed. Examples of processed meats are hot dogs, ham, bacon, salami, sausages, and lunch meats.

Sugar is thought, by some people, to feed cancer. That's not true. Eating too much non-nutritive sugar and refined, simple carbohydrates can cause an increase in insulin-like growth factor (IGF), which signals cells to grow. IGF is normal and necessary in the body. However, too much IGF is not good. First of all, limit your intake of sugar–no soft drinks, no bakery products, basically no junk food. Try to stay away from processed foods, period. Stay away from refined sugars. Stay away from simple carbohydrates that turn into sugar quickly in your body, like white bread, cookies, candy, and jams. Secondly, increase your intake of complex carbohydrates in the forms of whole grains, fruits, vegetables, beans, and legumes.

Fats can be a somewhat complicated topic. A diet high in saturated fat has been shown to help promote several diseases, one of which is cancer. A diet low in saturated fat and high in unsaturated fat has been shown to actually protect against several diseases, including cancer. This is another way of saying eat vegetables, not meat!

Fats are essential to our bodies, and omega-3s are listed in the Foods To Enjoy section, but a low-fat diet goes hand in hand with fighting cancer. Try to keep your fat intake to no more than 20% of your total daily food intake.

Fats to avoid are dairy products (other than skim or nonfat), margarine, lard, animal fats (except fish), and vegetable oils (except olive and canola oils). That means avoid most baked goods and snacks, unless they are healthfully made.

Omega-6s are also considered EFAs (essential fatty acids), but eating omega-6s is a balancing act because some omega-6s are bad for you when consumed in excess. This is primarily true for linoleic acid, found in many vegetable oils. U.S. diets tend to be too high in omega-6 fats, because we have a tendency to eat too much junk food. A healthy diet containing significant amounts of foods rich in omega-3 fats and omega-6 fats is necessary for good health, but the ratio should be close to 3:1 omega-6s to omega-3s. Ratios in the U.S. can be as high as 50:1! Is it any wonder that we're in the middle of a cancer epidemic? Avoid proinflammatory, refined and hydrogenated omega-6s that are found in vegetable oils such as corn, soy, sunflower, and safflower, and margarine. You can get omega-6s through olive oil, almonds, soybeans, and walnuts, but again, balance is everything with omega-6s.

Salt has been found to promote stomach and liver cancer—especially through eating salt-preserved, salted, or salty foods, according to the Second Expert Report published by the American Institute for Cancer Research and The World Cancer Research Fund. Their recommendation is less than 2 grams of sodium a day from all foods. Read food labels, try not to exceed 2,000 mg. (2 grams) of sodium per day. That equals a little less than one teaspoon of salt. Also, the USDA recommends that people who are 51 years of age or older, African American, and/or have high blood pressure, diabetes, or chronic kidney disease should not exceed 1500 milligrams per day.

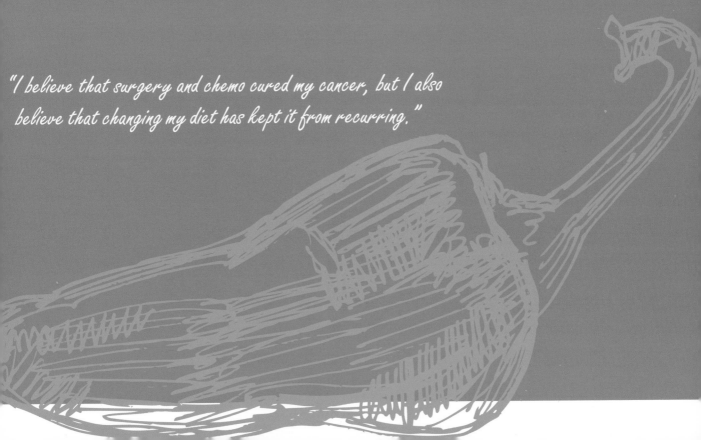

"I believe that surgery and chemo cured my cancer, but I also believe that changing my diet has kept it from recurring."

Cancer Fighting and Food Preparation Tips

Artificial Sweeteners are something I avoid. Although initial studies on many of them have proven that they do cause cancer in rats, further studies have shown that they do not cause cancer in humans. Studies still continue, and I don't want to take a chance. We are used to, especially in this country, eating foods that are overly sweet. I try to eat naturally and have become used to—and now favor—foods that are not too sweet. Why take a chance? Who knows what the next study will show?

Garlic contains many substances which have been and are still being studied for their anti-cancer effects. However, cooked garlic has been shown to lose its possible cancer-fighting properties. Get in the habit of crushing, mincing, or chopping your garlic first, then go about preparing the rest of your recipe. Allowing the crushed garlic even ten minutes to rest enables the garlic to hold on to its possible anti-cancer properties through cooking.

Grilling and firing up the BBQ is something we all love to do. However, cooking meats on high heat produces carcinogenic compounds called HCAs (heterocyclic amines). HCAs have been shown to cause cancer. This is true for not only red meats but chicken and fish also. It is not true for fruits and vegetables as they do not produce HCAs. Grill up the fruits and veggies to your heart's content, but avoid meats on the grill. If you're really set on slapping meat on the grill, here are some safety tips for grilling that will reduce your cancer risk:

Avoid flare-ups from fat dripping on the grill, you can do this by:

- Using a less fatty meat or fish.
- Keeping a spray bottle with water next to the grill and dousing the flare-ups as they happen.
- Not placing the meat/fish directly on the grill but rather on a piece of foil that has a few holes poked in it.
- Using a marinade. Marinating meat or fish prior to grilling has been shown to greatly reduce the production of HCAs.
- Not charring or burning the meat (flipping the meat/fish often helps).
- Using a smaller portion so it doesn't take as long to cook.
- Par-cooking the meat before placing it on the grill.
- Keeping the BBQ on low heat.

Onions have been shown to help fight cancer, but a recent study takes it a step further—the stronger tasting onions have more antioxidants than the milder tasting ones. Shallots, Western Yellow, New York Bold, and Northern Red have a stronger taste and a higher level of antioxidants. Empire Sweet, Western White, Peruvian Sweet, Mexico, Texas 1015, Imperial Valley Sweet, and Vidalia have a sweeter taste and fewer antioxidants.

Oils vary greatly in terms of degree of unsaturated and saturated fats. I primarily use olive and canola oils, as they are two of the highest in unsaturated fats and lowest in saturated fats.

Pesticides are to be avoided as some have been shown to be carcinogenic. People who work with pesticides have a higher rate of certain cancers.

Physical activity and daily exercise is a necessity to stay healthy. The latest recommendation is half an hour a day of moderate to vigorous exercise. Exercise considered moderate includes walking and biking. Exercise considered vigorous includes swimming and racing. A good rule of thumb is called the "talk test." If you can talk normally, but not sing, then you are exercising at a moderate level. If you can only say a few words without taking a breath, you are exercising at a vigorous level. Get an exercise buddy and make it a routine.

Salads are great, but ditch the iceberg lettuce. Iceberg lettuce has become the norm for most restaurants to serve, but it is mostly water and has little nutritional value. Instead, try using hearty greens such as arugula, cabbage, spinach, kale, collard greens, mustard greens, or watercress.

Smoking is something that should be totally avoided. According to the National Cancer Institute, there are more than 7,000 chemicals in tobacco smoke, and at least 250 of those are known to be harmful. Of the 250 known harmful chemicals, 69 chemicals can cause cancer. There is no upside here—just don't!

Sugars include dextrose, fructose, fruit juice concentrates, glucose, honey, lactose, maltose, molasses, sucrose, sugar (both white and brown), syrup (both corn and maple). These are to be avoided or used in limited amounts. If you do indulge, eat them with some protein, fat, or fiber. When eaten this way, simple sugars are processed in your body in a more healthful way and produce less insulin. The best thing to do is try to avoid these sugars as much as possible. Some of my recipes do call for a limited amount of brown sugar, but I use natural/raw brown sugar, which is only slightly better than brown sugar. The natural brown sugar is produced from the first crystallization of sugarcane and is therefore less processed. Regular brown sugar is generally just refined white sugar that has had molasses added to it. Moderation is key. High fructose corn syrup should be avoided altogether.

Supplements have not yet been proven to help fight cancer. The jury is still out on this topic; not enough data has been gathered. Some high-dose supplements may actually increase cancer risk. This is a personal choice and should be made after some research and a conversation with your doctor. Food probably remains the best source of vitamins and minerals.

Tanning Beds have been shown to probably cancer in humans. Run—do not walk!—in the opposite direction. Do not use them!

Tea of all types contains antioxidants. White and green teas are less processed than black tea, and they contain more antioxidants. Research is mixed on tea helping to prevent cancer. In laboratories, tea has been proven to fight cancer, but in human studies the results have been mixed. I gave up coffee when I was diagnosed and switched to green tea. It's not unusual for studies to be mixed. I'd rather err on the side of caution. If it hasn't been proven to harm me, it just might help me.

Vegetables are great, but their cooking methods can be a bit confusing. According to a recent study the Brassica vegetables, which are broccoli, Brussels sprouts, cauliflower, and green cabbage, have been shown in laboratories to help fight cancer. But new studies have found that boiling seriously depletes these vegetables of their cancer fighting properties. A better way of preparation is steaming, stir frying, or microwaving them.

In studies, green beans, beets, and garlic have been found to keep their antioxidant levels after most cooking methods, and artichokes were found to be the only vegetable that retained its high antioxidant level during all the cooking methods.

Vitamin D may have positive effects on fighting some cancers. Vitamin D is obtained through skin exposure to the sun, through supplements, and through diet, though few foods provide Vitamin D. Salmon, sardines, mackerel, and cod liver oil contain Vitamin D, along with fortified foods such as milk and cereals. The Vitamin D discussion is one you should have with your doctor as recommended Vitamin D levels vary according to gender and age.

Many doctors now believe that the current recommended amounts are insufficient and are recommending more. Sun exposure is one of the best ways to get Vitamin D, but several factors decrease the body's ability to make Vitamin D including dark skin, age (older people have impaired conversion in their skin to produce Vitamin D), heredity, obesity, and certain medications. Increasing exposure to the sun increases the risk of skin cancer, but using a sunscreen blocks Vitamin D synthesis in the skin. It's all a bit confusing, and—quite frankly—who knows for sure? There does not seem to be a definitive answer here. That's why some personal research and a discussion with your doctor would be advised.

How to Get There From Here

I work full time, and I don't have any household help. I have rearranged my life and my kitchen to accommodate my new way of eating. As I stated earlier, more time will be spent in the kitchen preparing, so if you can get your kitchen and yourself organized, a lot of time can be saved, and the end result will be productive and positive. I spend two to three hours every week, usually on a Sunday, in the kitchen cooking and preparing to set myself up for the week. If you have plenty of time on your hands, changing your eating habits and food preparation habits shouldn't be a problem, but if not...

Start by going through your refrigerator and cupboards. I know this is hard to do. However, the old stuff has to be replaced with newer healthier stuff eventually. So start by throwing out, giving away, or weaning yourself off the bad stuff. Slowly start replacing the bad foods in your cupboards and refrigerator with healthier choices.

Here are some suggestions for making your kitchen a healthier, cancer-fighting space:

- Read food labels for fat content. You want to avoid saturated fats such as butter, lard, palm oil, partially hydrogenated oils, and full fat dairy products.

- Read food labels for salt content. You'll be shocked to see how much salt is in prepared foods. The goal is to limit your total daily salt intake to about one teaspoon.

- Read food labels for sweeteners. Avoid any sweetener that isn't natural, such as artificial sweeteners, along with corn syrup, high fructose corn syrup, white sugar, and agave syrup.

- Start substituting white flour products with whole wheat products.

- Get rid of all processed meats. Meat that has been smoked, cured, or salted has been shown to cause cancer. Although it's tasty, cutting out processed meat is one of the most important steps you can nutritionally take to prevent cancer.

- Make room in your freezer, as it is going to become your best friend through this diet plan. Get rid of the junk and make room for the good stuff. Your freezer will make it possible to always have a healthy home cooked meal at your fingertips.

- Cut up fresh fruit, portion it out, and freeze it in snack-size freezer bags. Having fruit cut up ahead of time is great for blending up healthy, tasty smoothies.

- Make a larger portion when cooking main dishes and freeze half of it. A lot of the recipes in this book will serve 6-8 people. Most recipes freeze great and then you've got your work done for the upcoming week. Make the larger recipe and bag the leftovers in freezer bags for later enjoyment.

- Make or buy pizza dough and have it ready to go. Pizza dough freezes fine and is the basis for a really easy, quick dinner. Have a marinara sauce in the pantry for the sauce.

- Have a stockpile of beans and rice. Cans are okay without added salt or unhealthy oils. Rice, beans, and a salad is a quick, easy dinner when you're on the run.

- Make lunchtime salads for the week on Sunday. If you're using hearty greens, they will easily last the week in the refrigerator. Just leave off the dressing until you're ready to eat your salad.

- Buy an insulated lunch bag if you don't have one and a freezer ice pack. Start taking your lunch with you if you work. The lunch out of your new lunch box is going to be healthier (and less expensive) than lunch from a restaurant or food court.

- Plant some herbs. If you have a yard, great. If not, some pots on the balcony work just fine for most herbs. If you live in a cold climate, even if you have the herbs for part of the year during the warmer months, it's better than not having them at all. Plant oregano and basil, and put them in your salads.

- Buy berries on sale during the summer months and bag and freeze them for later use.

- Chop up any basil left on your basil plant before the weather gets cold. Mix it with olive oil and garlic and freeze it in plastic storage containers or freezer bags. It's great as a pizza sauce or over pasta during those cold winter evenings.

- If eating hot cereal, cook your breakfast cereal on Sunday also. Kept in an airtight container, it will last for several days.

- Try baking a loaf of bread. It's not as hard or time consuming as you might think. Slice it up all at once and put the slices in a freezer bag and put in the freezer.

- Sauté any leftover vegetables in a little bit of olive oil and put in freezer bags and freeze for later enjoyment on a pizza. Most vegetables taste great on a pizza. It cuts down any food waste, and it also cuts down on prep time on pizza day.

- Cook a casserole, such as *Lasagna* or *Mexican Cornmeal Casserole*, and cut it up into individual portions. Wrap the portions in small freezer bags and put them in the freezer for an easy, last minute dinner.

Before You Begin

Before you dive into the recipes in this book, here is some supplemental information and tips you should take a look at. This section includes guides for preparation and other important facts that will aid you in getting the most out of the cancer-fighting recipes you choose to prepare.

Blending hot liquids can be a dangerous process. The contents can explode from the pressure building up and blow the top off of the blender, spraying hot liquid all over the kitchen and all over you. The safest way is to allow the liquid to cool in the refrigerator overnight, but that isn't always possible. Here are some tips for blending hot liquids safely:

- Never fill the blender carafe more than half full.
- Use as slow a speed as possible.
- Remove the feed tube from the top of the blender to allow air to escape while blending and to prevent pressure build-up.
- Cover the lid with a dry kitchen towel.

Breads can vary in baking time depending on your oven. Here are a few tips to check if your loaf is done:

- Check the color of the crust, it should be a golden brown.
- Tap the loaf, it should sound hollow.
- Test the temperature using a digital read thermometer or meat thermometer, it should read 190 - 200 degrees F.
- Insert a toothpick or a sharp knife into the middle of the bread at the thickest part, it should come out clean and dry.

Canned and Jarred Foods are convenient, but be careful when buying them. Read the labels to ensure that they do not contain unhealthy oils, added sugars, or extra preservatives. Also look for low-sodium or no-sodium cans or jars.

Flour is generally ground from wheat, and the traditional all-purpose white flour has the germ and bran milled out and, in many cases, bleached. I like to use a white whole wheat flour instead. This is readily available in most grocery stores. It is a true whole wheat flour and still contains the bran and the germ, but it is made with white wheat instead of red wheat, so it is lighter in texture and more closely resembles all-purpose flour. If you can't find white whole wheat flour, use regular whole wheat flour and all-purpose flour at a ratio of 50/50.

Herbs are best when fresh, which is what I always use, since they are readily available from my garden. I do recommend, if possible, planting a few fresh herb plants, especially basil and oregano. If that is not possible, you can substitute dried herbs. The general rule of thumb is 3 parts fresh is equal to 1 part dry, or 1 tablespoon of fresh is equal to 1 teaspoon of dried.

Meats generally are to be avoided, but there are very few recipes in the cookbook that call for, or give the option of adding white meat chicken or turkey. Buy poultry that is free-range and 100% organic to ensure that you are getting the healthiest poultry available. Cook meats slowly using a low heat. Avoid grilling or using extreme temperatures they can cause the formation of carcinogenic compounds.

Microwaves are safe to use. According to the American Cancer Society they emit a low-frequency radiation that does not have enough energy to directly damage DNA. There is no evidence to suggest that microwaves cause cancer or make food radioactive. Always use microwave-safe containers. The safest thing to use is glass or ceramic containers.

Pizza is most easily made with a pizza paddle. Pizza paddles can be bought relatively inexpensively. If you don't own a pizza paddle, you can still make a great pizza by putting the rolled-out dough onto a cooling rack large enough to fit the pizza and then putting the cooling rack into the oven. Also, I don't use a pizza stone in my recipes. I find the pizza comes out great putting it directly on my oven rack. In the summertime, you can also use the grill!

Yeast can be added directly into dry ingredients, both active dry and instant (also known as fast acting or fast rising). It may also be dissolved in water before mixing. The temperature of the water will vary depending upon the chosen method. If adding yeast directly to dry ingredients, water should be 120-130 degrees F. If dissolving the yeast in water first (to give the yeast a little head start) water should be 110-115 degrees F. Although both methods are acceptable, I usually use the old-school method of dissolving the yeast first, as I find that produces a better loaf.

Yogurt Cheese is nothing more than yogurt with the whey (or liquid) drained out of it, which is what is the popular Greek yogurt actually is. A lot of companies that produce Greek yogurt are taking shortcuts and, instead of taking the time to drain the whey out of the yogurt, they are using thickening agents and preservatives. You can substitute Greek yogurt if you can find one without additives, but it's easy to make your own.

Kitchen Staples

These are the staples in my kitchen and pantry. I like to have these supplies on hand for easy, quick meal making. I generally have my herbs fresh, but that's not always convenient, so I recommend keeping dried herbs on hand.

Pantry Staples

- Almonds
- Almond butter
- Balsamic vinegar
- Beans (dried or canned)
- Broth (low-fat chicken or vegetable)
- Brown rice
- Canola oil
- Fruit spread (no sugar added)
- Lentils
- Oatmeal
- Olive Oil
- Raisins
- Raw brown sugar
- Red wine
- Refried beans (nonfat vegetarian)
- Spices (dried)
    - Cinnamon
    - Cumin
    - Curry
    - Oregano
    - Turmeric
- Tomatoes (canned)
- Walnuts
- Whole wheat flour
- Whole wheat pasta
- Whole grain bread
- Whole grain, unsweetened cereal

Refrigerator Staples

- Berries (fresh and frozen)
- Eggs
- Corn tortillas
- Dark chocolate
- Fresh garlic
- Fruit (fresh and frozen)
- Greens
    - Kale
    - Spinach
    - Collard
    - Mustard
- Herbs (fresh)
    - Basil
    - Cilantro
    - Oregano
    - Parsley
- Honey
- Milk (nonfat or soy)
- Pizza dough
- Tahini
- Tomatoes (fresh)
- Vegetables (all)
  Especially these, for soups/stews
    - Onions
    - Carrot
    - Celery
- Yeast
- Yogurt (plain, nonfat)

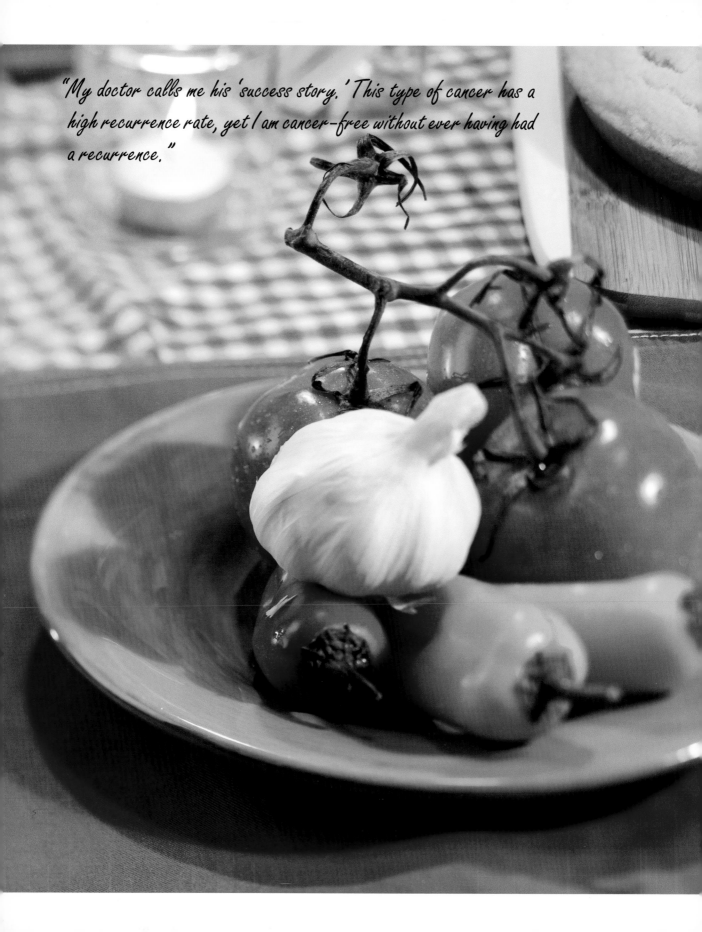

"My doctor calls me his 'success story.' This type of cancer has a high recurrence rate, yet I am cancer-free without ever having had a recurrence."

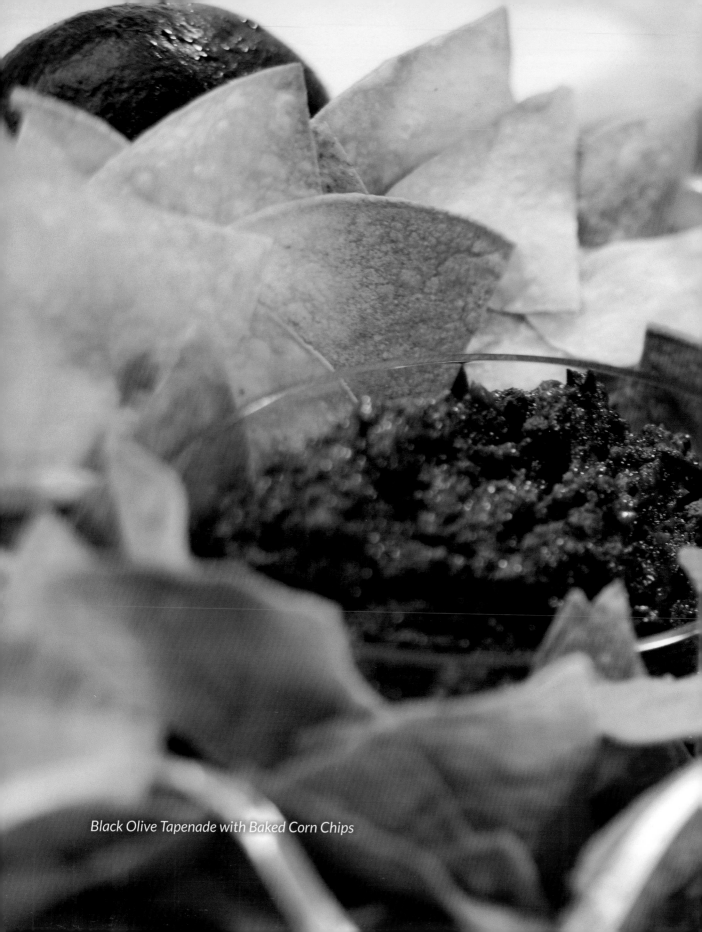

Black Olive Tapenade with Baked Corn Chips

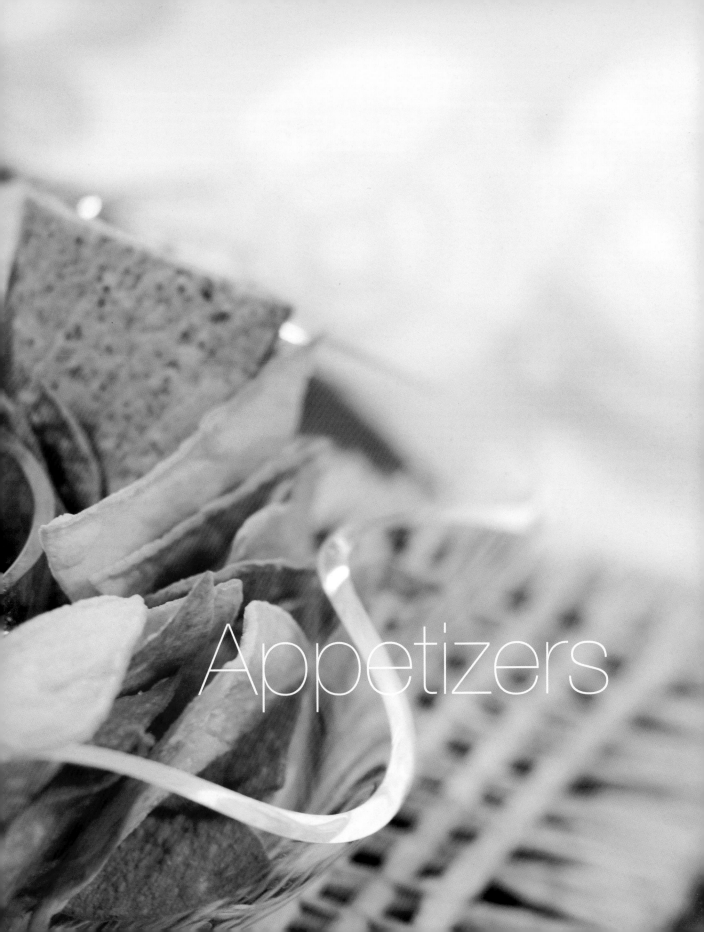

Appetizers

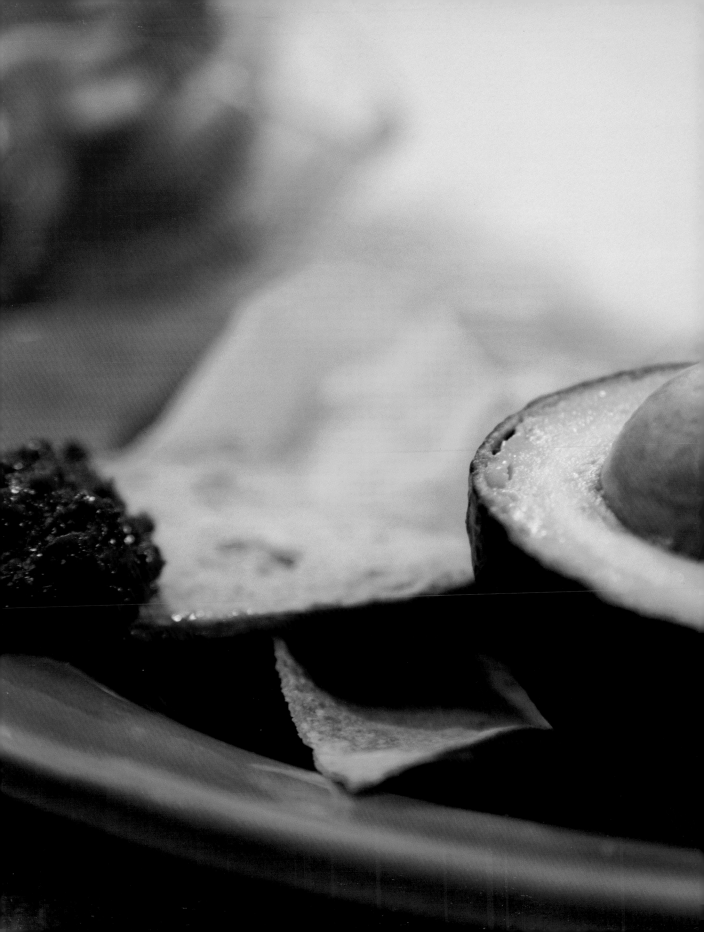

If you're having some friends over to visit, appetizers are great to serve when guests first arrive and the conversation is just getting going. A tasty appetizer sets the stage for your main meal. I like to make them up ahead of time before guests come over to give me more time to sit and enjoy the food and my friends. But they're not just for company. Appetizers make perfect snacks for you and your family even when you're just sitting around watching television.

Many times, the appetizers we are most accustomed to eating are made with unhealthy fats, deep-fried or laden with salt, all of which you want to avoid. But they don't have to be. If you keep it simple with healthy ingredients, you can still get raves on the yummy food and keep yourself, your family, and your friends on the avoid-cancer path.

Tomatoes, olives, beans, garlic, olive oil, eggplant, and spinach are all tasty and can be made into great appetizers. You can even make your own healthy chips! I guarantee that with eating these goodies, your friends will be slow to leave, and when they do finally depart, they will want to take the recipes home.

Baked Corn Chips

Corn chips don't have to be bad and forbidden. These chips don't take long to cook, they're not laden with the unhealthy oils that are known to help cause cancer, and they taste better than the ones you'll get in a store. As a matter of fact, once you've had these, the store-bought ones won't compare!

20 corn tortillas	Salt
Canola oil spray	Ground cumin (optional)

Cut each tortilla into quarters and layer pieces on a canola-oil sprayed baking sheet. Spray lightly with canola oil and season with salt and cumin.

Bake at 350 degrees F until crisp and brown. These taste great served warm, but they'll also hold up well for a couple of days of snacking.

Note: In a hurry for some quick munching? Place a corn tortilla in the microwave for 2 minutes, and you've got an almost instant healthy chip!

Makes 80 chips

Baked Whole Wheat Lavash Chips

Lavash is an Armenian unleavened flat bread. It's readily available in most of the supermarkets in Los Angeles. If you're lucky, it is also accessible near you.

These are a tasty healthy alternative to store-bought chips. They're easy to make and taste way better than anything you can get in the store.

1 package whole wheat lavash	Salt
Olive oil spray	Ground cumin

Preheat oven to 350 degrees F. Cut lavash into 2 inch squares and place on ungreased cookie sheet. Spray chips with olive oil spray. Then sprinkle with cumin and salt.

Bake on cookie sheet in oven until chips are crispy and brown, about 10 minutes.

Serve with *Hummus* or *Black Bean Dip* and enjoy!

Serves 6-8

Black Bean Dip

Black beans are simply a miracle food. Research has found that the darker the bean's seed coat, the higher the level of antioxidants. Therefore, black beans were found to have the most antioxidants of all beans. This is a tasty, guilt-free dip.

1 (16 ounce) can black beans, drained (save ¼ of the liquid)
½ cup salsa (mild or hot—your choice)
1 tablespoon balsamic vinegar
1 tablespoon olive oil
Juice of 1 lime

1 clove garlic, minced
¼ cup chopped cilantro
¼ cup chopped flat-leaf parsley
Salt and pepper
Crushed red pepper flakes to taste (optional)

Place all ingredients (except salt, pepper, and red pepper flakes) in a food processor and blend until smooth. Salt and pepper to taste. Add red pepper flakes if desired. Serve with *Baked Corn Chips*, *Whole Wheat Pita*, or raw vegetables.

Serves 3-4

Black Olive Tapenade

This is a great appetizer for a get together. Black olives contain anthocyanins, pigments which are high in antioxidants. In addition, according to the National Cancer Institute (NCI), studies show an association between an increased intake of garlic and a reduced risk of certain cancers.

2 cans or 3 cups olives, pitted and drained (the better the olives used, the more complex the taste)

2 large cloves garlic, minced
2-3 tablespoons olive oil
Black pepper

Combine all ingredients (except black pepper) in a food processor and pulse. Leave some texture (don't pulse until smooth). The olives should appear finely chopped and a little chunky. Add pepper to taste. Drizzle a bit more olive oil over the mixture before serving. The tapenade lasts for a good week in the refrigerator and can be doubled or tripled for a larger group of company. Serve with *Baked Corn Chips* or *Baked Whole Wheat Lavash Chips*.

Serves 4-6

Bruschetta

Studies conducted with tomatoes (high in the antioxidant lycopene) show that they appear to be very beneficial for fighting many different types of cancer. Basil and garlic have also shown in studies to fight the monster. You can't lose on any level with this appetizer—so good and so good for you!

4 cups tomatoes, chopped
¼ cup chopped fresh basil
3 cloves garlic, minced
¼ cup extra-virgin olive oil

Salt and pepper
Olive oil spray
1 whole wheat or whole grain baguette, cut in ¼ inch diagonal slices

Combine tomatoes, basil, garlic, and olive oil in a large bowl and mix well. Salt and pepper to taste. Place in the refrigerator and allow to cool for at least one hour to allow the flavors to meld. When ready, preheat the broiler or grill. Lay out the bread slices on a baking sheet and spray with olive oil. If using the broiler, place the sheet under the broiler and toast until slightly brown. If using the grill, place the bread slices directly on the grill and cook until slightly brown. You can serve the *Bruschetta* on top of toasted bread slices or separately in a bowl and let friends and family dip in for themselves.

Serves 3-4

Cucumber Yogurt Sauce

1 cup plain nonfat yogurt
½ cucumber, peeled and seeded
¼ cup chopped fresh cilantro
1 small tomato, seeded and diced
½ teaspoon raw brown sugar
Salt and pepper

Place all ingredients into food processor except tomato, salt, and pepper. Blend until smooth. Spoon in diced tomato. Salt and pepper to taste. Serve cold.

Roasted Red Pepper

I roast my red peppers directly on my outdoor grill. It's easy. Just place the washed red pepper directly on the grill, turn your peppers as needed until the skin has turned black and starts to blister. When the pepper skins have turned black, remove the peppers from the grill, place them into a bowl, and cover. You can also put the peppers in a paper bag and tightly close the bag. Whichever method, steam the peppers in an air-tight container for about 15 minutes.

After you remove the peppers, the black skin will peel off easily. Discard the skin along with the seeds.

If you don't have a grill, you can also roast the peppers on a cookie sheet by broiling until black and blistered or by placing the peppers directly on your stove top burner. Make sure you turn frequently and watch closely!

Once roasted, the peppers can be frozen and used later in other recipes. They freeze and thaw out great!

Roasted Red Pepper Dip

Bell peppers are excellent sources of Vitamins A and C. This is a nonfat version of an old favorite.

1 tablespoon olive oil
2 cloves garlic, minced
½ red onion, chopped
2 roasted red peppers, chopped
1 tablespoon balsamic vinegar

½ cup plain nonfat yogurt
½ cup nonfat sour cream
2 teaspoons chopped fresh basil
Salt and pepper

Heat olive oil in a skillet. Add garlic, onion, and red peppers and cook for 2 minutes, stirring frequently. Add vinegar and cook for about 10 more minutes or until most of the moisture is out of the pan and the onions have some color.

Transfer ingredients into a bowl and refrigerate until cool. Add the rest of the ingredients (except salt and pepper) and stir well. Salt and pepper to taste. Serve with *Baked Corn Chips* or raw veggies.

Serves 3-4

Garbanzo Bean Croquettes with Cucumber Yogurt Sauce

Garbanzo beans are members of the legume family. High in antioxidants, protein, minerals, and fiber, they are low in fat and a good source of folate, which has been shown in studies to help fight colorectal cancer.

1 can garbanzo beans (chickpeas), drained and rinsed
1¾ cups Panko bread crumbs, divided
8 ounces fresh mushrooms
1 small tomato, seeded and diced
1 small onion, diced finely

1 clove garlic, minced
2 tablespoons chopped flat-leaf parsley
1 teaspoon cumin
Salt and pepper
Canola oil spray

Preheat oven to 350 degrees F. Mix garbanzo beans, ¼ cup Panko bread crumbs, mushrooms, tomato, onion, garlic, parsley, and cumin in a food processor until well blended. Salt and pepper to taste. Place the remaining 1½ cups Panko bread crumbs into a bowl. Spoon rounded tablespoons of the croquette mixture into the Panko bread crumbs and coat on all sides. By hand, flatten into flat, round silver dollar shapes, about 2 inches in diameter and place on a canola oil-sprayed cookie sheet. Spray croquettes with canola oil and then bake in oven for 45 minutes or until done. The outside should be crispy.

Serve Croquettes hot, with cold *Cucumber Yogurt Sauce*

Serves 4-6

Eggplant and Roasted Red Pepper Caviar

Red peppers are rich in phytochemicals that help fight cancer, and they rank among the top ten foods that contain several antioxidants, including beta-carotene and lutein. Eggplant is usually considered a vegetable, but it's actually a fruit. Eggplants are members of the nightshade family, as are tomatoes and potatoes, and are rich in phytochemicals such as monoterpene, which possess certain cancer-fighting properties. This is a versatile sauce that can be used as a dip for crackers or corn chips or served over sautéed veggies or grilled polenta. If desired, use a jar of roasted red peppers instead roasting your own. You can also use chopped fresh red peppers without roasting them, although the extra layer of flavor from the roasting really adds to this dish.

1 large eggplant, peeled and chopped into cubes
3 tablespoons olive oil
1 large onion, chopped
2 large tomatoes, chopped

1 green bell pepper, chopped
4 *Roasted Red Peppers*, chopped
4 cloves garlic, crushed
Salt and pepper
1 tablespoon balsamic vinegar

Lightly salt the eggplant cubes and let sit for about 30 minutes to remove some of the liquid in the eggplant. Then rinse and pat dry with a paper towel. Heat the olive oil in a large skillet over medium heat. Add the onion and cook until the onions are soft. Add the patted dry eggplant cubes along with the remaining ingredients to the pan with the cooked onions. Stir well and continue to sauté on high until vegetables get some color. Reduce heat, cover, and simmer until all ingredients are soft. Turn heat on high for the last couple of minutes, stirring constantly, until most of the remaining water is out of the vegetables. Mash together well.

Salt and pepper to taste.

Serves 4-6

Stuffed Mushrooms

Ordinary button mushrooms are low in calories and high in nutrition. Studies have shown that these mini gems may help fight breast cancer and prostate cancer.

8-12 ounces of white button mushrooms or cremini mushrooms
3 large cloves of garlic, minced
1 medium onion, diced finely
4 cups of spinach leaves, chopped
¼ cup quick oats
1 tablespoon olive oil
1 tablespoon chopped flat-leaf parsley
1 tablespoon chopped fresh oregano

1 teaspoon chopped fresh thyme
1 medium tomato, finely chopped
Salt and pepper
3 tablespoons low-fat grated Parmesan
½ cup shredded cheese (part-skim mozzarella, veggie, or soy)
Olive oil spray
Crushed red pepper flakes to taste (optional)

Grilled Marinated Artichokes

The little artichoke is an antioxidant giant! One of the highest ranked foods in antioxidants per serving.

3 large artichokes or 6 baby artichokes, trimmed and cleaned
¼ cup balsamic vinegar
¼ cup extra-virgin olive oil
1 large clove garlic, minced
1 tablespoon Dijon mustard
Juice of 1 lemon
¼ teaspoon salt
¼ teaspoon pepper

Cover the bottom of a large pot with an inch of water and place the artichokes in the pot. Bring water to a boil. Reduce heat to a simmer, cover, and cook until artichokes are par-cooked. When done, remove from pot and allow to cool. Split in half lengthwise and remove hairy choke. Set aside.

Prepare marinade by whisking all the other ingredients in a bowl. Dip each artichoke half into the marinade and then place cut side down in a 9" x 13" baking dish. After all have been dipped, pour remaining marinade over them, cover, and allow to sit in the refrigerator for 2 hours to overnight.

Place artichokes on medium-hot grill. Cook for about 5-10 minutes on each side to create grill marks. Serve warm with *Garlic Dip*.

Serves 5-6

Garlic Dip

¼ cup nonfat sour cream
¼ cup plain nonfat yogurt
1 clove garlic, minced
Juice of ½ lemon
1 teaspoon raw brown sugar
Pepper to taste

Whisk together and chill until ready to serve.

Preheat oven to 400 degrees F. Clean mushrooms by wiping them off with a damp towel and remove the stems. Mince the stems. Spray a medium skillet with olive oil spray and place over medium-high heat. Add the onion and mushroom stems. Sauté quickly until onions are translucent, about 5 minutes. Reduce heat to medium low and add the remaining ingredients, except the cheese and salt and pepper. Add red pepper flakes if desired. Salt and pepper to taste. Spray a cookie sheet with olive oil and place the mushrooms cap side up on the sheet. Generously stuff the mushrooms with the spinach mixture. Sprinkle a little Parmesan cheese over the top of each mushroom, then top with a small amount of shredded cheese. Place cookie sheet in preheated oven for about 20 minutes. Serve hot.

Serves 3-4

Healthy Layer Dip

I like this for a special occasion, like the Super Bowl or the Oscars. Gotta have some good munchies for those special times! It's a healthier version of a fat-laden favorite.

1 (16 ounce) can fat-free refried beans
8 ounces plain nonfat yogurt or
nonfat sour cream
8 ounces salsa (red or green)
1 avocado, diced
1 large onion, diced
1 large red pepper, diced

1 large yellow pepper, diced
1 cup cooked, diced chicken breast (optional)
¼ cup chopped black olives
2 bunches chives, chopped
1 small bunch of cilantro, chopped
1 cup shredded cheese (part-skim mozzarella, veggie, or soy)

In a large skillet, sauté onion and peppers until onion is translucent but not totally soft. Both vegetables should still have a bit of crunch. Set aside. On an 11" dinner plate, spread out the refried beans, covering the plate. On top, spread the yogurt or sour cream and then the salsa. Layer the remaining ingredients atop the salsa, including the cooked onions and peppers, leaving the cheese for last. Serve with *Baked Corn Chips*.

Serves 5-6

White Bean Dip

This bean dip is tasty and practically fat-free.

2 cans white beans, partially drained
1 teaspoon cumin
2 teaspoons freshly squeezed lemon juice
3 cloves garlic, coarsely chopped
1 tablespoon sesame tahini
1 handful flat-leaf parsley
1 handful cilantro
Salt and pepper
Crushed red pepper flakes (optional)

Place all ingredients (except salt and pepper) in food processor until smooth. Add crushed red pepper flakes to taste if desired. Salt and pepper to taste. Serve with *Baked Corn Chips*, *Whole Wheat Pita*, or raw vegetables.

Serves 4-6

Hummus

Hummus makes a great appetizer, snack, or spread.

1 (16 ounce) can of garbanzo beans (chickpeas), include 1/2 of liquid
Juice of one lemon
1 tablespoon tahini
2 cloves garlic, minced
1 tablespoon olive oil
1 handful cilantro
Salt and pepper

Place all ingredients, except salt and pepper, in a food processor and blend until smooth. Salt and pepper to taste. Add red pepper flakes if desired. Serve with *Baked Corn Chips*, *Whole Wheat Pita*, or raw vegetables.

Serves 3-4

Spinach Dip

This is a low-fat version of the classic. Spinach is a nutritional powerhouse that is high in fiber, minerals, vitamins, omega-3 fats, and phytochemicals: flavonoids and carotenoids. Many recent studies have shown that the phytochemicals in spinach help to prevent several chronic illnesses, including cancer. Add onions and garlic to the mix and you've got not only a delicious appetizer, but a commanding combination of cancer-fighting foods.

1 (8-ounce) package frozen chopped spinach, thawed and drained
1 medium ripe avocado
1 cup plain nonfat yogurt
¼ cup nonfat sour cream
2 tablespoons extra-virgin olive oil
½ cup flat-leaf parsley

½ cup cilantro
1 bunch green onions
1 tablespoon balsamic vinegar
1 clove garlic, minced
4 teaspoons prepared horseradish
Salt and pepper

Place all ingredients in a food processor (except salt and pepper) and blend until thoroughly mixed. Chill for at least 2 hours before serving, allowing the flavors to meld together. Salt and pepper to taste. Serve with *Baked Corn Chips*, *Whole Wheat Pita*, or raw vegetables.

Serves 4-6

Hummus is so flexible— you are only limited by your imagination!

Try adding these:

Crushed red pepper flakes

6 cloves of roasted garlic.

One fire roasted red pepper

½ cup spinach

4 large, softened sun-dried tomatoes.

Green Pea and Avocado Dip

This is a slightly lighter version of guacamole. Avocado is pretty high in fat and calories. Adding green peas reduces fat and gives this dish its own special flavor.

1 cup frozen peas, thawed
1 large avocado, pit and skin removed
1 large clove garlic
1 tablespoon olive oil
¼ cup plain nonfat yogurt
Juice of 1 lime

1 tablespoon soy sauce
¼ cup chopped flat-leaf parsley
1 tomato, finely chopped
¼ cup chopped cilantro + extra for sprinkling
Salt and pepper

Place all ingredients (except tomato, one tablespoon chopped cilantro, salt and pepper) in a food processor and blend until smooth. Stir in chopped tomatoes. Salt and pepper to taste. Sprinkle the remaining cilantro on top.

Serves 3-4

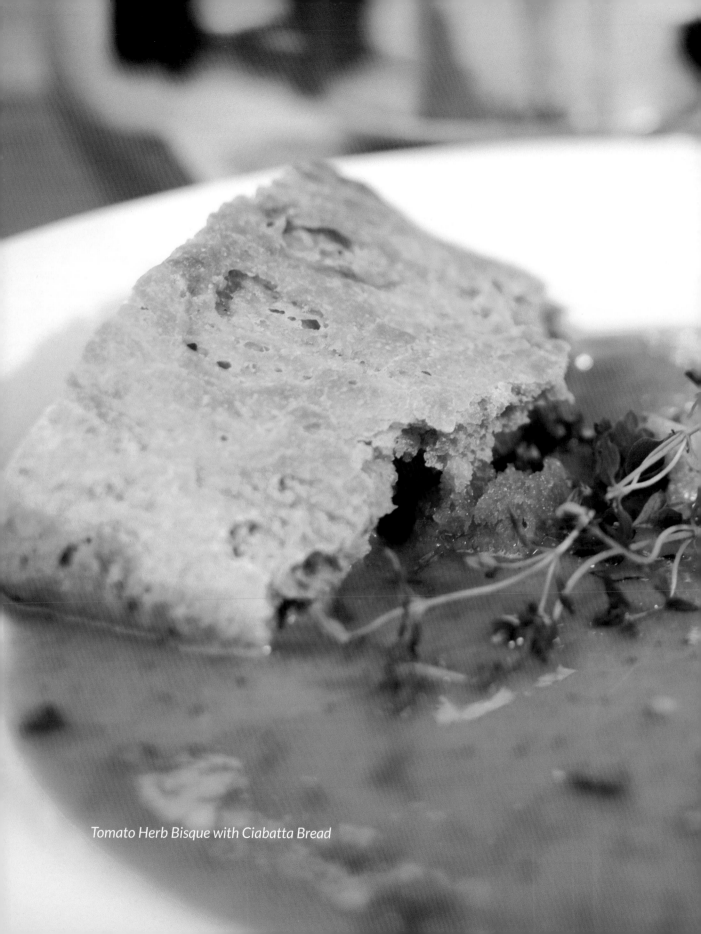

Tomato Herb Bisque with Ciabatta Bread

Soups

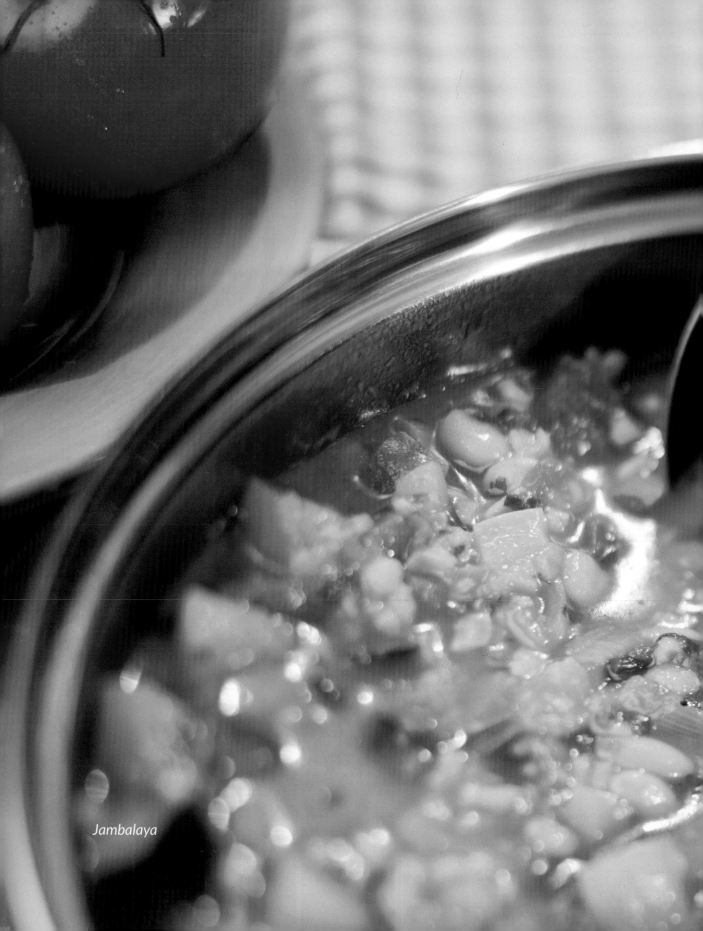

Jambalaya

You don't need to be laid up in bed with a cold to enjoy a steaming hot bowl of soup or a nice chunky stew. Soups and stews can be warm and comforting on a winter's evening, but most of us don't think of them as a complete meal. Chock full of tasty and healthy ingredients, though, many of them can be.

Soups and stews are relatively inexpensive to make, and they usually freeze well. I normally double the recipe and freeze half. Then, when I get home from work, I have a nutritious meal waiting for me to just heat up. They're also pretty easy to prepare, because we're talking about a one-pot dish.

Easy, inexpensive, convenient, and healthy—soups and stews are a mainstay.

Black Bean and Brown Rice Soup

Beans and rice are very nutritious and together are considered a complete protein. Serve with *Garlic Bread* or toasted corn tortillas.

6 cups vegetable or nonfat chicken broth
½ pound dried black beans
1 small onion, chopped
½ cup red pepper, chopped
½ cup green pepper, chopped
½ cup celery, chopped
½ cup carrots, chopped
2 cloves garlic, minced
2 tablespoons olive oil
1 (16 ounce) can diced tomatoes

1 (16 ounce) can pinto beans, undrained
1 cup cooked brown rice
1 tablespoon Worcestershire sauce
(organic, no high-fructose corn syrup)
2 bay leaves
1½ teaspoons ground cumin
½ cup chopped fresh cilantro
½ cup chopped fresh flat-leaf parsley
Crushed red pepper flakes to taste
Salt and pepper

Rinse black beans well. In a large saucepan, combine vegetable broth and beans. Bring to a boil and then simmer for 5 minutes. Remove from heat and cover. Let beans soak in broth for 1 hour. In a large skillet, sauté onions, peppers, celery, carrots, and garlic in olive oil until semi-tender. Add to beans and broth mixture after the beans have soaked for one hour. Add tomatoes and pinto beans and bring to a boil. Reduce to a simmer, cover, and cook for about 2 hours. Add cooked rice, Worcestershire sauce, bay leaves, cumin, cilantro, parsley, and red pepper flakes (if desired) and continue to simmer until rice and beans are tender. Mash slightly to thicken soup. Salt and pepper to taste.

Serves 6-8

Cabbage Soup

A good friend of mine makes this with kielbasa. Loving the taste, but wanting to avoid the processed meat, I have altered the recipe to be equally as good without the meat, with that great, savory taste.

3 quarts vegetable or nonfat chicken broth
2 large potatoes, unpeeled and diced
16 ounces sauerkraut, drained well
1 large onion, diced
2 large unpeeled apples, diced
½ head small cabbage, diced in 1 inch pieces
2 tablespoons raw brown sugar
4 large cloves garlic, chopped

1 tablespoon dried marjoram
3 tablespoons chopped fresh oregano
½ teaspoon allspice
1 tablespoon paprika
1 tablespoon olive oil
Crushed red pepper flakes (optional)
Salt and pepper to taste

In a stockpot, cook onions in oil until soft. Add other ingredients. Simmer until vegetables are tender.

Serves 6-8

Split Pea, Potato, and Leek Soup

This is a traditional favorite, and for good reason. Peas are high in fiber, protein, and low in fat. They are also a good source of protein, folate, and vitamins A and C.

1 tablespoon canola oil
1 onion, chopped
3 carrots, chopped
3 stalks celery, chopped
1 leek bottom (white part only), rinsed well and chopped
2 cloves garlic, crushed
1 pound dried yellow split peas, rinsed
1 medium russet potato, unpeeled, and chopped

10 cups vegetable stock
1 medium sweet potato, peeled and chopped
1 cup kale, chopped
2 bay leaves
½ cup flat-leaf parsley, chopped
½ cup cilantro, chopped
1 teaspoon dried thyme
Salt and pepper

In a large stockpot over medium-high heat, sauté the oil, onion, carrots, celery, leek, and garlic until onions are translucent, about 10 minutes. Add remaining ingredients. Bring to a boil, reduce heat to low, and partially cover. Simmer for 2 hours, stirring occasionally until peas dissolve and soup thickens. Remove bay leaves. Using a hand-held electric blender, blend until semi-smooth. This soup should be a little chunky. Serve with a dollop of nonfat sour cream and enjoy!

Serves 6

Indian Spiced Lentil Soup

Lentils are cousins of the bean and packed with protein, fiber, and complex carbohydrates.

8 cups vegetable broth
2 cups tomato juice
¾ cup brown lentils
¾ cup lentils (preferably orange)
1 large yellow onion, diced
3 stalks celery, diced
2 large carrots, shredded
2 cloves garlic, crushed

2 tablespoons balsamic vinegar
2 tablespoons tomato paste
2 teaspoons ground turmeric
2 teaspoons ground cumin
2 teaspoons curry powder
1 cup kale, finely chopped
¼ cup chopped flat-leaf parsley
Salt and pepper

Combine all of the ingredients in a large stockpot, except kale and parsley. Mix well and bring to a boil. Reduce heat to a simmer. Cover and allow to cook for 1 hour or until vegetables are tender and lentils are soft. Add kale and parsley. Stir well to combine. Cook for another 20 minutes. Salt and pepper to taste. Serve with *Whole Wheat Pita Bread* or *Not So Flat Garlic Flat Bread* and enjoy!

Serves 6-8

No Cream of Asparagus Soup

No cream. No kidding. You'll never miss it. This soup is rich and wonderful without it.

2 tablespoons olive oil	2 medium carrots, cut in thirds
2 pounds fresh asparagus, ends trimmed	2 cups cauliflower florets
	¼ cup fresh chopped flat-leaf parsley
1 pound fresh mushrooms, sliced	1 tablespoon dried thyme
1 large onion, diced	1 tablespoon dried basil
4 cloves garlic, minced	1 bay leaf
6 cups vegetable or fat-free chicken stock	1 cup cold, nonfat milk
	1 tablespoon cornstarch
4 stalks celery, cut in thirds	Salt and pepper

Cut 1 inch tips off of asparagus. Set the stems aside for later. Heat 1 tablespoon of the olive oil in a skillet over medium heat and add mushrooms and asparagus tips. Cook until water is removed from mushrooms and asparagus tips are tender. Set aside.

Heat remaining 1 tablespoon of olive oil in a large stockpot over medium heat and add onions and garlic. Cook until onions have some color (about 10 minutes). Add vegetable stock and all the other vegetables, including the asparagus stems, and herbs. Bring to a boil, reduce heat to low, and simmer until all vegetables are tender.

Remove bay leaf and allow soup to cool. Puree in electric blender in batches and pour back into pot (please see safe blending instructions under Before You Begin). Bring soup back to a boil.

Dissolve cornstarch in milk. Whisk the cornstarch mixture into the boiling soup, whisking constantly to avoid lumps. Remove soup from heat. Add cooked mushrooms and asparagus tips. Stir well. Salt and pepper to taste.

Serves 4-6

Note: This soup does not freeze well. It becomes very thin after freezing, so it is best eaten fresh.

No Cream of Broccoli and Mushroom Soup

Got a taste for a nice creamy, thick soup on an autumn afternoon? This soup will satisfy without being laden with the fat that's in most cream soups.

1 large onion	3 large garlic cloves, peeled
1 large leek, cleaned and trimmed	2 tablespoons olive oil
3 carrots, cut in thirds	1 bunch broccoli, in ½ inch pieces
3 stalks celery, cut in thirds	1 pounds mushrooms, sliced
1 small bunch flat-leaf parsley	1 cup nonfat milk
1 bunch broccoli, rough chopped	½ cup plain nonfat yogurt
½ cauliflower, rough chopped	½ cup nonfat sour cream
7-8 cups vegetable or	2 tablespoons cornstarch
fat-free chicken broth	Salt and pepper

Place onion, leek, carrots, celery, parsley, 1 bunch rough chopped broccoli, cauliflower, and garlic cloves in a large stockpot. Add the broth to the pot, just covering the vegetables. Depending on the size of your vegetables, you will use 7-8 cups. Bring broth and vegetables to a boil. Lower heat, cover, and simmer for 1 hour or until all vegetables are very tender. Set aside until cool.

Sauté sliced mushrooms and remaining chopped broccoli in olive oil until tender and all of the water is out of the mushrooms. Salt and pepper to taste. Set aside.

Puree broth mixture in batches in an electric blender until completely blended. (Please see safe blending instructions under Before You Begin). Transfer each carafe of blended soup to a second large soup pot, until all boiled vegetables and broth have been blended.

In a medium bowl, mix together the milk, yogurt, sour cream, and cornstarch. Whisk together until well blended.

Bring the soup to a boil and quickly whisk in the cornstarch mixture. Add sautéed broccoli and mushrooms. Simmer for ½ hour, stirring often. Salt and pepper to taste. Serve hot.

Serves 6-8

Note: This soup does not freeze well. It becomes very thin after freezing, so it is best eaten fresh.

Vegetarian Chili

This is a thick, rich chili full of veggies and flavor. You won't miss the meat but you will gain a ton of vitamins and nutrients from the myriad veggies in this dish. I've served this at parties and even my meat loving friends love it. No one has ever asked me, "Where's the beef?" It takes a bit of time to make because of the chopping involved, but it lasts for while in the refrigerator, freezes great, and is well worth the effort.

3 tablespoons canola oil
2 small stalks celery, chopped
2 medium carrots, diced
1 large onion, chopped
1 small green pepper, chopped
1 small red pepper, chopped
1 small poblano pepper, chopped
2 yellow summer squash, diced
2 zucchini, diced
1 cup spinach, chopped
½ pound mushrooms, chopped
1 (15 ounce) can white beans, undrained
1 (15 ounce) can black beans, undrained
1 (15 ounce) can cannelloni beans, undrained

1 (15 ounce) can kidney beans, undrained
1 (15 ounce) can garbanzo beans, undrained
2 (28 ounce) cans whole peeled tomatoes
2 (28 ounce) cans diced tomatoes
32 ounces tomato juice
3 cloves garlic, crushed
¼ cup tomato paste
½ cup chopped flat-leaf parsley
¼ cup chopped fresh cilantro
2 tablespoons chili powder
2 tablespoons cumin
Salt and pepper
Crushed red pepper flakes (optional)

In a large stockpot, heat canola oil. Add all vegetables and garlic and sauté for about 10 minutes until vegetables are tender. Stir in all other ingredients (except salt and pepper) and bring to a boil.

Reduce heat and simmer until vegetables are tender, about 45 minutes. Add red pepper flakes if desired. Salt and pepper to taste.

Serves 6-8

Curry Lentil Stew

This is a filling meal, with the consistency falling somewhere between a soup and a stew.

2 tablespoons olive oil
1 large onion, diced
4 carrots, diced
4 stalks celery, diced
3 cloves garlic, minced
4½ cups water
1 cup green lentils

1 cup lentils (preferably orange)
1 (14.5 ounce) can crushed tomatoes
1 (14.5 ounce) can diced tomatoes
¼ cup chopped flat-leaf parsley
2 teaspoons curry powder
4 cups fresh spinach, chopped
Salt and pepper

In a medium saucepan, heat olive oil over medium heat. Add onion, carrots, celery, and garlic. Sauté until the vegetables have some color, about 10 minutes. Stir in water, lentils, canned tomatoes, parsley, and curry. Bring to a boil, then cover and reduce to simmer for 1 hour or until thick. Add spinach last and stir until well mixed. Cook for 10 minutes more. Salt and pepper to taste.

Note: Lentils soak up liquid. If stew gets too thick, add another of can of diced or crushed tomatoes.

Serves 4-6

Lentil, Spinach, and Kale Soup

Lentils are high in protein, fiber, and iron. They make this soup a real winner!

2 tablespoons olive oil
1 onion, diced
2 stalks celery, chopped
2 large carrots, chopped
2 cloves garlic, crushed
1 pound lentils (any kind) cleaned and rinsed
8 cups vegetable or nonfat chicken broth
1 (28 ounce) can peeled tomatoes, with juice

2 bay leaves
½ teaspoon curry
¼ teaspoon allspice
1 pound fresh spinach, julienned
3 large kale leaves, julienned
½ cup chopped fresh flat-leaf parsley
Salt and pepper

In a large stockpot, sauté onion in oil until soft. Add celery, carrots, and garlic. Sauté until all vegetables have some brown color. Add remaining ingredients, except spinach, kale, and parsley. Bring to a boil, reduce heat, and simmer until lentils are tender, about 1 hour. Add the spinach, kale, and parsley, and cook for another 20 minutes. Salt and pepper to taste. Serve hot and enjoy!

Serves 4-6

Jambalaya

This dish requires some chopping, but it's well worth it. What a tasty treat this is and it is jammed packed with healthy vegetables. The poblano pepper gives it enough of a kick for me, but if you really like things spicy, some hot sauce can be added to taste. White meat turkey or chicken can also be added if desired.

This dish makes a nice Sunday night supper, or serve it at your next party for an unexpected crowd pleaser.

3 tablespoons canola oil
1 stalk celery, chopped
1 small onion, chopped
1 large carrot, diced
2 cloves garlic, crushed
1 small green pepper, chopped
1 small red pepper, chopped
1 small poblano pepper, chopped
1 small yellow summer squash, diced
1 small zucchini, diced
1 bunch green onions, chopped
1 (28 ounce) can peeled tomatoes
8 cups vegetable broth
1 (14 ½ ounce) can white beans, undrained

1 cup brown rice, uncooked
¼ cup chopped fresh basil
¼ cup chopped flat-leaf parsley
¼ cup chopped fresh cilantro
1 tablespoon Cajun seasoning
1 teaspoon dried thyme
1 teaspoon paprika
1 bay leaf
1 small jalapeño pepper with seeds removed, chopped finely (optional)
1 pound white meat turkey or white meat chicken, cooked and diced (optional)
Salt and pepper

Heat oil in a large stock pot. Add celery, onion, carrots, garlic, peppers, and sauté for about 5 minutes until vegetables are semi-tender. Stir in all other ingredients (except salt and pepper) and bring to a boil. Reduce heat and simmer until rice is tender, about 1 hour. Salt and pepper to taste.

Note: You might need more liquid depending on the size of the vegetables you use and once the rice soaks up the liquid. Add extra vegetable broth if needed.

Serves 6-8

Lentil Stew

Lentils are high in fiber, protein, and antioxidants. They are low in calories, fat, and are cholesterol free. There is nothing bad to say about lentils. To top it off, they're inexpensive, filling, and taste great. Lentils are simply good stuff, and this stew is an excellent way to add them to your diet.

1 tablespoon olive oil
1 russet potato, unpeeled and diced
1 large onion, diced
4 carrots, diced
4 stalks celery, diced
3 cloves garlic, minced
7 cups vegetable stock
2 cups tomato juice
1½ cups green lentils
1½ cups red lentils
1 (28 ounce) can whole tomatoes, broken up

1 (8 ounce) can tomato sauce
1 (15 ounce) can sweet corn, drained
1 tablespoon raw brown sugar
2 teaspoons fresh thyme, chopped
3 bay leaves
½ cup chopped flat-leaf parsley
3 tablespoons dehydrated onions
2 tablespoons garlic powder
1 teaspoon paprika
1 teaspoon celery salt
Salt and pepper

Heat the oil in a medium saucepan over medium-high heat. Add onion, potato, carrots, celery, and garlic. Sauté until vegetables get some color, about 10 minutes. Stir in vegetable stock, tomato juice, tomato sauce, lentils, canned tomatoes, corn, brown sugar, thyme, bay leaves, parsley, dehydrated onions, garlic powder, paprika, and celery salt.

Bring to a boil, reduce heat to a simmer, and cover. Simmer for 1 hour until thick. Salt and pepper to taste.

Note: If you don't serve this dish immediately, more liquid will have to be added, as the lentils soak up the liquid and the stew will get too thick. If needed, thin out to your desired consistency with vegetable stock, chicken stock, or tomato juice. Any of these liquids will work, however the tomato juice will give it a stronger tomato flavor.

Serves 6-8

Pinto Bean Soup

Pinto is Spanish for "blotchy or marked," which obviously refers to the pinto beans' variations of color.

16 ounces dried pinto beans
11 cups vegetable broth
2 tablespoons olive oil
1 large onion, finely chopped
3 large carrots, chopped
2 large stalks celery, chopped
2 red peppers, chopped
3 garlic cloves, minced
¾ cup brown rice, uncooked

1 (15 ounce) can fat-free refried beans
4 cups chopped greens
4 large tomatoes, diced
½ cup chopped fresh cilantro
½ cup chopped fresh flat-leaf parsley
2 tablespoons ground cumin
1 tablespoon balsamic vinegar
Salt and pepper

Rinse and clean beans well. Place beans in large stockpot with 4 cups of broth. Bring to a boil and boil for 3 minutes. Cover, remove from heat, and let stand for 1 hour. Sauté onion, carrot, celery, red peppers, and garlic in olive oil until vegetables begin to get some color, about 10 minutes. Add sautéed vegetables to soaked beans. Add all other ingredients (except salt and pepper). Cover and cook on a low heat until vegetables and beans are tender, about 1 hour. Salt and pepper to taste.

Serves 8

Refried Bean Soup

The refried beans make a great, thick, rich base for this soup, and the flavor will surprise you.

1 large onion, finely chopped
3 large carrots, chopped
2 large stalks celery, chopped
3 cloves garlic, minced
2 tablespoons olive oil
4 cups vegetable broth
1 (14.5 ounce) can fat-free refried beans

1 (28 ounce) can black beans (in liquid)
1 (15 ounce) can sweet corn, drained
1 (28 ounce) can peeled tomatoes with juice
½ cup chopped fresh cilantro
½ cup chopped fresh flat-leaf parsley
2 tablespoons ground cumin
Salt and pepper

Sauté onion, carrots, celery, and garlic in olive oil until vegetables begin to get some color, about 10 minutes. Combine refried beans and 2 cups of vegetable broth in blender and blend until smooth. Combine with all other ingredients. Cook until tender, about 30 minutes. Salt and pepper to taste.

Serves 6-8

Ratatouille

This is a dish, just like a good chili, that's better the next day after the flavors have had a chance to meld. It not only looks appetizing with so many different colors in it but contains several cancer-fighting ingredients. I add beans to this dish for protein. Serve with brown rice and a nice garden salad. This recipe also freezes well, so I double it up and have it ready to go in the freezer for a quick dinner during the week.

2 small eggplants, cubed
2 tablespoons olive oil
1 large onion, diced
3 cloves garlic, crushed
1 zucchini, diced
1 yellow summer squash, diced
½ pound mushrooms, sliced
1 red pepper, diced in 1 inch chunks
1 orange pepper, diced in 1 inch chunks
1 green pepper, diced in 1 inch chunks
4 large tomatoes, diced
½ cup dry white wine

2 tablespoons tomato paste
2 bay leaves
½ cup white beans, canned or cooked fresh
½ cup black beans, canned or cooked fresh
¼ cup chopped fresh basil
½ teaspoon dried oregano
¼ teaspoon dried thyme
2 tablespoons chopped flat-leaf parsley
Salt and pepper

Lightly salt the eggplant cubes and let sit for about 30 minutes to remove some of the liquid. Then rinse well and pat dry with a paper towel.

In a large saucepan, heat olive oil over medium heat. Stirring constantly, add onions and cook for about 10 minutes until onions begin to have some color. Add garlic, eggplant, zucchini, squash, mushrooms, and peppers and cook for 15 minutes, stirring occasionally, until all of the water has cooked out of the mushrooms and the eggplant. Add tomatoes, white wine, tomato paste, and bay leaves. Cook for another 5-10 minutes, stirring occasionally until all of the ingredients begin to get mushy. Add the beans, spices, and herbs. Salt and pepper to taste.

Cook for a couple of minutes more, stirring constantly, and remove from heat.

Serves 6-8

Southwestern Black Bean and Brown Rice Chili

Rice and beans make a complete protein and the Southwestern flavors are delicious. Spice it up if you like it with a kick of jalapeño, or prepare it with less fire. Either way it's great and great for you, and you can never go wrong with beans. This is a large recipe but freezes great for later enjoyment.

1 pound dried black beans, rinsed
4 cups water
8 cups vegetable broth
2 tablespoons olive oil
1 large onion, finely chopped
1 poblano pepper, finely chopped
1 carrot, shredded
2 large stalks celery, finely chopped
1 cup kale, finely chopped
4 cloves garlic, minced
1 bunch green onions, chopped
1 (28 ounce) can peeled tomatoes with juice
2 tablespoons ground cumin

1 teaspoon ground oregano
2 tablespoons chili powder
½ teaspoon cayenne pepper
Crushed red pepper flakes (optional)
1 jalapeño pepper, finely chopped (optional)
1 cup plain nonfat sour cream (optional)
Juice of 2 limes
1 bunch chopped fresh cilantro
1 cup brown rice, uncooked
1 (15 ounce) can sweet corn, drained
Salt and pepper

In a large stockpot, bring beans and water to a boil over high heat. Cover, reduce heat, and simmer for 45 minutes. Beans will still be a bit hard but will have absorbed most of the water. Add 4 cups vegetable broth and continue simmering for 1 hour.

While beans are cooking, sauté onions, pepper, carrots, celery, kale, garlic, and green onions in olive oil until tender.

Remove 2 cups of the bean mixture and puree in blender. (Please see safe blending instructions under Before You Begin.) Return the blended mixture to the pot along with the sautéed vegetables. Add the peeled tomatoes, breaking them apart as you add them into the pot. Add spices, lime juice, cilantro, rice, and corn. Cover and simmer over low heat until rice is thoroughly cooked and most of the liquid is absorbed, about 1½ hours. Salt and pepper to taste.

Serve with *Garlic Bread* and/or a dollop of nonfat sour cream and enjoy!

Serves 6-8

"Scarborough Fair" Spiced Lentil Soup

I call this the "Scarborough Fair" soup because every time I go out to the garden to pick the herbs for this soup I sing to myself, "Parsley, sage, rosemary, and thyme..."

3 tablespoons canola oil
1 large onion, diced
3 cloves garlic, crushed
4 stalks celery, diced
4 large carrots, diced
4 potatoes, unpeeled and diced
1 pound dry lentils

12 cups vegetable or
fat-free chicken broth
3 tablespoons chopped fresh sage
3 tablespoons chopped fresh rosemary
3 tablespoons chopped fresh thyme
½ cup chopped flat-leaf parsley
Salt and pepper

In a large stockpot, sauté onion in oil until soft. Add garlic, celery, potatoes, and carrots and sauté until the vegetables have some brown color. Add remaining ingredients (except salt and pepper) and mix well. Bring to a boil, reduce heat, and simmer until all ingredients are mixed and lentils are tender, about 1 hour. Use an electric hand blender to roughly blend the soup. Don't blend till smooth. Leaving some lentils intact thickens the soup. Salt and pepper to taste.

Note: If you don't serve this soup immediately, more liquid will have to be added. The lentils soak up the liquid and the soup will get too thick. If needed, thin out with vegetable or fat-free chicken stock.

Serves 8

Soupili

I love this cross between a soup and chili! It's better if made the day before and eaten on day two after the flavors have had a chance to meld. This recipe freezes very well for later use.

1 (19 ounce) can black bean soup
1 (15.5 ounce) can crushed tomatoes
1 (15.5 ounce) can diced tomatoes
2 (15.5 ounce) cans black beans
1 (15.5 ounce) can vegetarian chili
1 (15.5 ounce) can pinto beans
1 (15.5 ounce) can garbanzo beans (chickpeas)
1 cup carrots, diced

1 cup onions, diced
1 cup celery, diced
3 cloves garlic, minced
2 tablespoons chili powder
1 tablespoons cumin
½ cup chopped fresh flat-leaf parsley
½ cup chopped fresh cilantro
2 cups white meat chicken (optional)

Puree the black bean soup. Pour into a large stockpot along with all of the other ingredients (no need to drain the cans of beans). Bring to a boil, then lower heat and simmer for 2 hours, stirring occasionally.

Serves 6-8

Squash and Carrot Soup

This soup tastes so rich and creamy, you'll never know it's fat-free! There's no cream or butter in this recipe, but it tastes as thick and as rich as if there were. To add to its charm, this dish couldn't be easier to prepare. Just put all the ingredients in the pot, cook it, and blend it! You'll find this colorful soup warm, filling, and flavorful. The nut topping makes this dish special enough to even serve to company.

1 large onion, quartered
2 large carrots, cut in half
4 large stalks celery, cut in half
1 large butternut squash, peeled and cut in large chunks (actually any winter squash can be used here)
3 cloves garlic
1 bunch flat-leaf parsley
5-6 cups vegetable broth

Dash of nutmeg
Salt and pepper
¼ cup raw almonds, finely chopped
¼ cup unsalted sunflower seeds, finely chopped
¼ cup finely diced apple
2 tablespoons finely diced chives
2 tablespoons finely diced raisins

Place onion, carrots, celery, squash, garlic, and parsley in a large stockpot. Add just enough of the vegetable broth to barely cover the vegetables. Bring to a boil. Reduce heat, cover, and simmer until all vegetables are soft, about 45 minutes. Turn off heat. Puree in batches in an electric blender until completely blended (please see safe blending instructions under Before You Begin). Return mixture to the pot, and season with salt, pepper, and nutmeg to taste.

Make a topping by mixing together in a small bowl almonds, sunflower seeds, apple, chives and raisins. Top each bowl of soup witha large spoonful of topping.

Serves 5-6

Tomato Herb Bisque

This soup couldn't be any easier to make. Everything just gets plunked into a blender and pureed. My next door neighbor declared, "That tomato soup was the best soup I ever had in my life!" Fresh herbs make this soup a winner.

The taste is gourmet, but the preparation couldn't be simpler. Tomatoes are a carotene-rich food, and studies confirm that eating more carotene-rich foods will reduce not only your risk of cancer, but also your risks of heart disease, hypertension, and stroke.

2 (14 ounce) cans fat-free chicken broth or vegetable broth
1 (15 ounce) can garbanzo beans, undrained
1 (15 ounce) can pinto beans, undrained
1 large red pepper, quartered
1 large orange pepper, quartered
1 (15 ounce) can diced fire roasted tomatoes
1 (15 ounce) can crushed tomatoes
¼ cup chopped curly parsley
¼ cup chopped flat-leaf parsley
¼ cup chopped fresh basil
¼ cup chopped fresh cilantro
1 large clove garlic, chopped
1 tablespoon fresh oregano
1 tablespoon balsamic vinegar
2 tablespoons raw brown sugar
1 cup nonfat milk
3 tablespoons cornstarch
1 small hot pepper, diced, seeds removed (optional)
Salt and pepper

This soup is a bit unusual, as it gets blended first, then cooked. All of the ingredients will not fit into one blender carafe, so you will have to fill twice. Place ½ of the broth, garbanzo beans, pinto beans, and red pepper into a blender and puree until the mixture is smooth (with hot pepper if desired). Pour into a soup pot.

Place the remaining broth, orange pepper, diced tomatoes, and crushed tomatoes, both types of parsley, basil, cilantro, garlic, oregano, and balsamic vinegar into blender and blend until mixture is smooth. Pour into soup pot. Add brown sugar. Bring soup to a boil, reduce heat, and simmer for 30 minutes.

In a small cup, dissolve cornstarch in milk. Bring soup back up to a boil and slowly whisk in cornstarch mixture. Soup will thicken slightly. Salt and pepper to taste. Serve hot.

Serves 6-8

Tomato Vegetable Soup

This soup is really thick and hearty with a lot of flavor. It has lots of good veggies and beans, both of which are powerhouse foods. It also freezes great for later use.

5 cups vegetable broth
4 large stalks celery, chopped
4 large carrots, diced
2 large onions, chopped
1 green pepper, chopped
1 red pepper, chopped
1 orange pepper, chopped
½ pound mushrooms, chopped
½ head cauliflower, chopped
2 (15 ounce) cans black beans, undrained
1 (15 ounce) can pinto beans, undrained

1 (28 ounce) can whole peeled tomatoes, broken up into smaller pieces
1 (15 ounce) can sweet corn, drained
1 (15 ounce) can fat-free refried beans
1 (28 ounce) can whole peeled tomatoes
1 cup flat-leaf parsley, chopped
3 cloves garlic, crushed
2 tablespoons Creole or Cajun seasoning (salt-free)
Salt and pepper

Pour the vegetable broth into a large stockpot. Add all of the ingredients to the broth, except one can of the whole tomatoes, the can of refried beans, parsley, garlic, and Creole or Cajun spice.

In an electric blender or food processor, blend together the can of refried beans and the second can of whole tomatoes. Add to the stockpot and mix well. Add the parsley, garlic, and Creole or Cajun spice. Bring the soup to a boil, then lower the heat and simmer for 45-60 minutes, until the carrots are tender. When the carrots are tender, the soup will be done. Salt and pepper to taste.

Serves 6-8

Chicken and Tomato Stew

2 tablespoons olive oil
1 large onion, chopped
1 cup celery, chopped
1 cup carrots, chopped
1 large leek bottom (white part only), rinsed and chopped
3 cloves garlic, minced
4 cups tomato soup (You'll need 4 cups ready-to-eat tomato soup, not condensed. You can also use my *Tomato Herb Bisque*)
2 cups vegetable broth
4 medium red potatoes, quartered

1 (15 ounce) can sweet corn, drained
1 cup frozen peas
1 cup red wine
1 (28 ounce) can tomatoes, broken up
½ cup fresh flat-leaf parsley, chopped
2 bay leaves
1 teaspoon dried thyme
1 teaspoon dried mace
2 cups fresh spinach, chopped
2 large chicken breasts, shredded
Salt and pepper

Vegetable and Apple Curry Soup

This is an interesting soup with an Indian flavor. In laboratory studies, both apples and curry have been shown to help prevent cancer growth.

3 tablespoons olive oil
1 medium onion, diced
1 large clove garlic, minced
1 large carrot, peeled and sliced
2 celery stalks, sliced
3 medium apples, with skin, cored and sliced
1 tablespoon curry powder
1 teaspoon turmeric
½ teaspoon fresh thyme
8 ounces butternut squash, peeled and cut in chunks

6 cups vegetable stock
½ small cauliflower, cut in chunks
½ cup nonfat sour cream or plain nonfat yogurt
1 cup nonfat milk
1 tablespoon cornstarch
2 cups cooked brown rice
¼ cup chopped fresh flat-leaf parsley
¼ cup chopped fresh cilantro
Salt and pepper

In a large stockpot, heat the oil over medium heat. Add the onion and sauté until the onion is translucent. Add the garlic, carrot, celery, and apples. Sauté until the vegetables are soft. Add the curry, turmeric, and thyme. Mix well. Add the vegetable stock, squash, and cauliflower. Bring the mixture to a boil and reduce the heat to a simmer and cook for another 45 minutes. Remove from heat. Puree in batches in an electric blender until completely blended. (Please see safe blending instructions under Before You Begin). Place back on the heat and bring to a boil. Dissolve cornstarch in milk. Add to the boiling soup mixture and stir well. Lower heat and simmer for 5 minutes. Soup should thicken a little. Add rice, parsley, and cilantro. Salt and pepper to taste. Serve hot.

Serves 6-8

Here's a healthy comfort food with lots of veggies, tomatoes, and garlic that's perfect for family dinner. Serve with a hot, toasty, whole grain baguette. Make it ahead—it freezes very well for later enjoyment.

In a large skillet, over a medium-high heat, sauté the onions, celery, carrots, leek, and garlic in olive oil until semi-tender and vegetables get some color. You will have to stir frequently to avoid burning. Add all other ingredients (except cooked chicken and spinach) and bring to a boil. Reduce to a simmer, partially cover (allow room for some air to escape), and cook for about 1 hour, stirring occasionally. Add cooked chicken and spinach. Continue to cook until all vegetables are tender, about one more hour. Remove bay leaves before serving. Salt and pepper to taste.

Serves 6-8

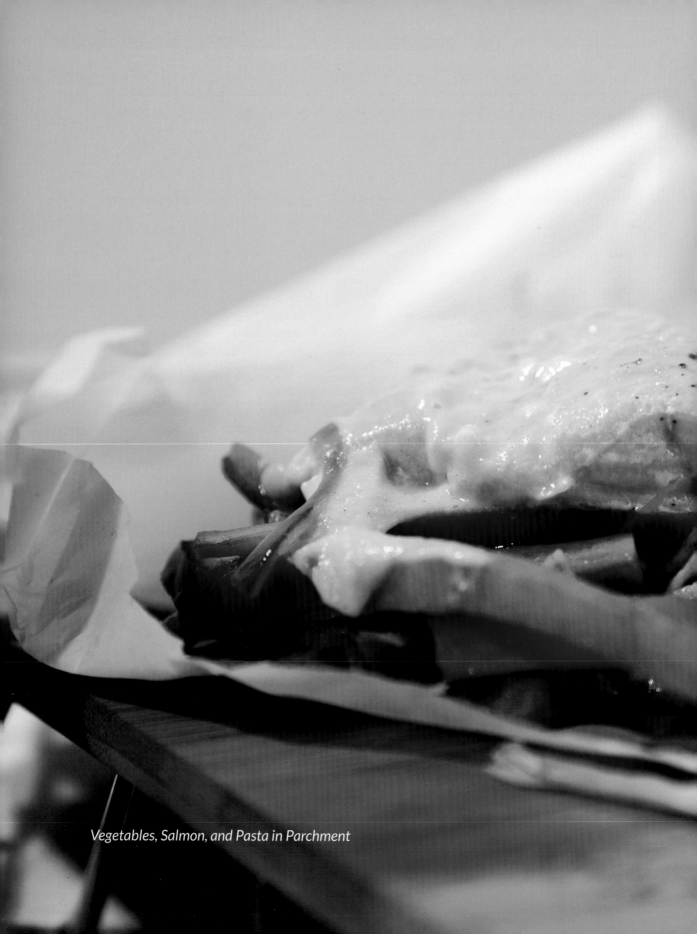

Vegetables, Salmon, and Pasta in Parchment

Main Courses

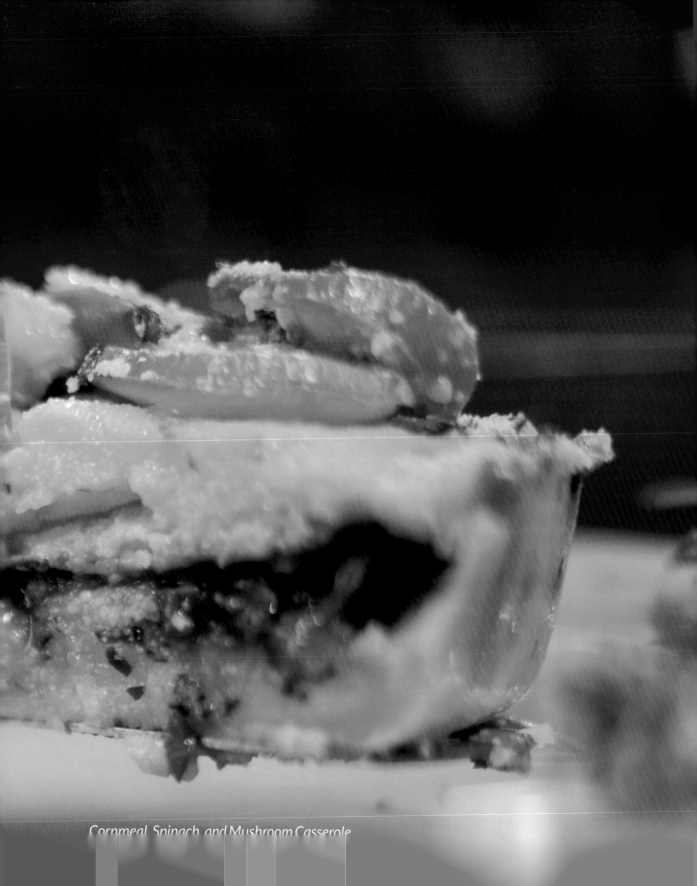

Cornmeal, Spinach, and Mushroom Casserole

I like to eat, and in terms of cooking, I like to experiment with different ethnic cuisines, so you'll find that the recipes in this section are literally all over the map.

The main ingredients in the bulk of these dishes are vegetables. As I've amended my diet to eat more healthfully, meats and heavy sauces have moved out of my culinary repertoire, and fresh vegetables, herbs, and appealing spices have moved in. Main courses composed of vegetables, whole grains, and fresh herbs—altogether a recipe for a healthy diet.

As you try out the recipes in this section, you'll find that healthy food doesn't have to mean boring food. When I entertain, I serve these dishes, and my guests always leave happy, satisfied, and—most times—requesting the recipes!

Indian Spiced Grilled Vegetable Skewers

Both cumin and turmeric have been shown to help fight cancer. The rub, once grilled, soaks into the veggies and creates a nice crust.

1 large zucchini, cut in 1 inch chunks
2 yellow squash, cut in 1 inch chunks
1 large onion, cut in 1 inch chunks
1 small eggplant, cut in 1 inch chunks
1 red pepper, cut in 1 inch chunks

½ pound button mushrooms
16 cherry tomatoes
Olive oil spray
¼ cup olive oil for brushing
Salt and pepper

Rub

1 teaspoon chili powder
1 teaspoon cumin
1 teaspoon coriander
1 teaspoon ground fennel
½ teaspoon cloves

1 teaspoon cardamom
1 tablespoon turmeric
3 tablespoons olive oil
¼ cup chopped cilantro

Mix all the ingredients of the rub in a small bowl to create a paste. Place vegetables into a large bowl and pour the rub over the vegetables. Combine well. Skewer the vegetables onto 4 skewers. Spray skewers with olive oil. Salt and pepper both sides. Place on a medium-hot grill and grill until the vegetables are tender, turning several times and brushing with olive oil while grilling. Serve over *Indian Spiced Brown Rice*. Top with *Curry Sauce*.

Journey Cakes with Black Bean Sauce

This is a fun, unusual supper—pancakes for dinner! Some historians believe these flat corn cakes were originally called "journey cakes" because in earlier times they could be carried on long trips in saddlebags and baked along the way. Remember, beans are a power food! Serve with a salad.

1 cup cornmeal
2 teaspoons baking powder
½ teaspoon salt
1 egg white
½ cup water

½ cup fat-free milk
1 tablespoon canola oil
½ cup canned sweet corn, drained
1 tablespoon pimento, chopped
Canola oil spray

Preheat griddle or large skillet to medium-high. Place all ingredients (except corn and canola oil spray) into a bowl and stir to combine. Once thoroughly mixed, add corn. Spray preheated griddle or skillet generously with canola oil and pour batter onto the griddle to form 4 inch pancakes. Cook on one side about 3 minutes, flip, and cook about another 2 minutes. Top with *Black Bean Sauce*.

Serves 4

Black Bean Burrito with Lime Dressing

Mexican food doesn't have to be a no-no when you're committed to eating healthfully.

1 (15 ounce) can black beans, drained
1 tomato, chopped
2 green onions, chopped
1 cup cooked brown rice
½ cup canned sweet corn, drained
¼ cup shredded cheese (part-skim mozzarella, veggie, or soy)

¼ cup chopped cilantro
Crushed red pepper flakes (optional)
4 large whole wheat tortillas
1 ripe avocado, mashed
¼ cup plain nonfat yogurt or nonfat sour cream
Salt and pepper

Lime Dressing

1 clove garlic, finely chopped
Juice of 1 lime
Zest of 1 lime

2 tablespoons olive oil
Salt and pepper

Preheat oven to 350 degrees F. Place beans, tomato, green onion, rice, corn, cheese, and cilantro in a large bowl and mix together well. Salt and pepper to taste. Add crushed red pepper flakes if desired. Place all of the ingredients for the lime dressing in a small bowl and whisk together well. Add dressing to bean mixture and spread down center of each tortilla. Fold sides in, roll to form burritos. Place on a baking sheet and bake in preheated oven for 15 minutes or more, until burritos are hot and cheese is melted. Remove from oven. Top with avocado and nonfat sour cream.

Serves 4

Bean Tostadas

4 corn tortillas
½ (15 ounce) can fat-free refried beans
¼ cup cooked brown rice
¼ cup enchilada sauce
10 pitted black olives
¼ cup shredded cheese (part-skim mozzarella, veggie, or soy)

½ cup shredded lettuce
½ cup diced tomatoes
Salsa (optional)
Mashed avocado (optional)
Nonfat sour cream or plain nonfat yogurt (optional)
Diced tomatoes (optional)

Preheat oven to 350 degrees F. Heat tortillas in oven until crisp. Spread refried beans over tortillas, top with rice and enchilada sauce. Crumble the olives over sauce. Sprinkle the shredded cheese on top. Place the tortillas in the oven for 5 minutes to melt cheese. Remove from oven and top with lettuce, tomatoes, and optional toppings. Serve with extra sauce for dipping.

Serves 4

Cornmeal, Spinach, and Mushroom Casserole

Polenta has been around for centuries and was originally known as a peasant food. Lately, at least in the U.S., it's being found in more and more gourmet recipes. Polenta is made out of cornmeal boiled in water to become a kind of porridge, so I'm calling a spade a spade and I've called this a cornmeal casserole. This is a fun casserole to serve to guests, because its layers look really pretty when sliced. It's a great way to get your spinach, too. Serve with your favorite pasta sauce (from a jar or homemade) along with a nice crisp salad. My favorite is an arugula salad.

2 tablespoons extra-virgin olive oil
1 large onion, chopped
3 large cloves garlic, crushed
1 pound cremini mushrooms, cleaned and sliced
½ cup dry red wine
6 large tomatoes, 3 sliced and 3 diced
2 tablespoons tomato paste
1 tablespoon chopped fresh rosemary
1 tablespoon chopped fresh thyme

4 cups fresh spinach, chopped
3 cups water
3 cups vegetable broth
2 cups cornmeal
¼ cup chopped flat-leaf parsley
½ cup shredded cheese (part-skim mozzarella, veggie, or soy)
¼ cup low-fat grated Parmesan cheese
Salt and pepper
Canola oil spray

Have all of your ingredients ready before you begin, because once you start working with the cooked cornmeal, you will have to work fast—it hardens quickly.

In a large skillet, heat the olive oil over medium-low heat. Add the onion and cook until the onion is soft. Add the garlic and mushrooms and sauté until the water is out of the mushrooms. Add the wine, diced tomatoes, tomato paste, rosemary, and thyme. Cook on high, stirring constantly until half of the liquid has evaporated (about 5 minutes). Add the spinach, stirring constantly until the spinach wilts into the mixture. Add more wine if necessary. Salt and pepper to taste. Set aside.

Preheat the oven to 375 degrees F. In a large pot, add the water and broth and bring to a boil. Lower the heat and then slowly whisk in the cornmeal, stirring constantly until it becomes a porridge consistency. Add the parsley. Salt and pepper to taste.

Work quickly when assembling the casserole. Spoon half the polenta into a canola oil-sprayed 9" x 13" baking dish. Smooth out the top of the polenta with a spatula. Spread the spinach, tomato, and mushroom mixture on top of the cornmeal evenly, using a slotted spoon to avoid spooning in too much liquid. Sprinkle cheese over the mixture. Sprinkle half of the Parmesan cheese on also. Pour the remaining polenta mixture over all, and carefully spread out to the sides of the casserole dish. Layer the top of the casserole with the sliced tomatoes and sprinkle the remaining Parmesan cheese over the top. Bake in preheated oven for 30 minutes, until the top is golden brown. Allow to cool for 10-15 minutes before cutting into squares.

Serves 6-8

Curried Bulgur-Stuffed Zucchini

Research is still being conducted on curcumin, a component of turmeric (and one of the spices in curry powder). Early studies have been positive, suggesting that people who eat turmeric-rich diets have lower rates of breast, prostate, lung, and colon cancers. Also worth looking at is the fact that the cancer rate in India, where turmeric is widely used, is much lower than ours in the U.S. (with the exception of tobacco related cancers). If you like Indian food, you should enjoy this dish. What a tasty and healthy way to use up the (usually prolific) zucchini in your summer garden!

2 large zucchini
Olive oil spray
½ teaspoon granulated garlic
¼ teaspoon salt
¼ teaspoon pepper
1 cup bulgur, uncooked
2 cups vegetable broth or fat-free chicken stock
1 teaspoon curry powder
1 tablespoon olive oil

1 small onion
3 cloves garlic, minced
1 leek (bottom white part only) rinsed well and diced
1 large tomato, diced
8 basil leaves, chopped
½ teaspoon cumin
¼ cup raisins
1 chicken breast, cooked without skin and shredded (optional)

Preheat grill or oven to medium-high, 350 degrees F. Slice the zucchini down the middle, lengthwise.

Scoop out the seeds down the middle of the zucchini to create a 'boat.' Spray the inside of the zucchini with olive oil. Sprinkle on the granulated garlic and salt and pepper. Place on the preheated grill, flesh down, to get those nice grill marks and cook on both sides until tender. If you don't have a grill, bake in preheated oven on a cookie sheet until tender. Remove from heat and allow to cool.

In a large saucepan, combine the bulgur, vegetable broth, and curry. Stir well and bring to a boil over a high heat. Reduce the heat to a simmer, cover, and simmer until the bulgur is cooked (about 20 minutes). Remove from heat. Salt and pepper to taste.

In a large skillet, combine the olive oil, onion, garlic, and leek. Cook over a medium heat until onions and leeks are soft. Add tomatoes, basil, cumin, and raisins and stir to combine well. Add the mixture to the bulgur and mix together well. If you are including the chicken breast, add the shredded chicken and combine well.

Stuff the zucchini by spooning the bulgur mixture down the center of the zucchini. Position the stuffed zucchini on a cookie sheet and place in preheated grill or oven for 10 minutes. Remove from oven. Serve hot, topped with *Curry Sauce*.

Serves 3-4

Curried Spinach and Lentils

I love Indian food, but all of the Indian cookbooks I've seen call for spices that I can't always find in my local markets. Turmeric, a seasoning commonly used in the traditional dishes of India, is readily available. A major plus—it has recently been discovered by western scientists to be quite possibly a miracle spice full of anti-cancer properties. Lentils are inexpensive, extremely nutritious, and in recent studies they have been shown to reduce the risk of breast cancer. This is my version of a spinach-lentil dish often served in Indian restaurants.

2 cups lentils (preferably a mix of yellow and red)
4 cups vegetable broth
1 teaspoon turmeric
1 teaspoon paprika
1½ teaspoons curry powder
2 teaspoons ground cumin
1 tablespoon light olive oil or canola oil
1 large onion, chopped finely

2 cups canned stewed tomatoes, broken up
8 ounces mushrooms, sliced
3 cloves garlic, minced
1 pound fresh spinach, chopped
Juice of one lemon
Salt and pepper
1 teaspoon fresh, finely chopped chili pepper
4 cups cooked brown rice

Mix all the lentils together and wash thoroughly. In a large saucepan, bring the vegetable broth to a boil and add the lentils, turmeric, paprika, curry, and cumin. Cover and simmer on a low heat until the lentils are soft and all of the liquid is absorbed, about 30 minutes.

While the lentils are cooking: in a large skillet, sauté the onion in the oil until the onions are translucent. Add the tomatoes, mushrooms, and garlic to the onions and cook until the mushrooms are soft. Add the spinach and cook until the spinach wilts, about 2 minutes. Add the juice of the lemon.

Using an electric hand held blender (or a potato masher), mash down the lentils, leaving some lentils intact. Add the onion-spinach mixture to the lentils and combine well. Salt and pepper to taste. Serve with brown rice. Top with *Marinated Tomatoes* (see below).

Serves 4-6

Marinated Tomatoes

2 large tomatoes, diced finely
2 cloves garlic, minced
3 tablespoons olive oil

3 tablespoons balsamic vinegar
Salt and pepper

Combine all ingredients in a bowl and mix well.

Vegetables, Salmon, and Pasta in Parchment

This is truly a fun meal! Everyone gets his or her own parchment bag with veggies, salmon, and pasta. It's a quick, fun way to prepare foods that will cook evenly at the same time. I've chosen these vegetables, but you can mix and match any veggies you choose for this dish as long as you don't choose vegetables that have a lot of water in them (like mushrooms). Even without salmon it's a great, fun dish!

4 (4 ounce) wild salmon fillets, skin removed
6 tablespoons extra-virgin olive oil
1 red onion, thinly sliced
2 cloves garlic, minced
1 red bell pepper, julienned
1 cup butternut squash, julienned
1 large carrot, julienned
1 cup snow peas
¼ cup Dijon mustard plus 2 tablespoons
1 cup chopped kale

4 cups cooked whole wheat pasta (preferably a short pasta, like penne)
¼ cup chopped flat-leaf parsley
2 tablespoons chopped fresh oregano
2 tablespoons chopped fresh basil
2 tablespoons low-fat grated Parmesan cheese
2 medium plum tomatoes, thinly sliced and patted dry
½ cup *Balsamic Vinegar Reduction*
Salt and pepper

Preheat oven to 400 degrees F. Salt and pepper the salmon fillets, set aside. Sauté the onion and garlic in 1 tablespoon olive oil until soft and set aside.

Place the bell pepper, squash, carrot, snow peas, kale, cooked onions, and garlic in a large bowl. Add 2 tablespoons olive oil, and ¼ cup of the Dijon mustard. Mix well until all veggies are coated. Salt and pepper to taste. Pour remaining 3 tablespoons olive oil onto pasta. Toss with Parmesan cheese, parsley, oregano, and basil.

Fold four 15-inch square pieces of kitchen parchment paper in half. One piece at a time, starting near the top of the fold, draw a half of a heart, using as much of the paper as possible, and ending at the bottom of the fold. Cut the heart shapes out along your drawn lines. Then open the heart shapes up and lay flat on a large surface. Place ¼ of cooked pasta on each sheet next to the fold, about ⅓ down from the top of the heart. Top with ¼ of the vegetable medley. Place a salmon fillet on top of vegetables of each packet. Spread the remaining 2 tablespoons of Dijon mustard split evenly over each piece of salmon. Place the sliced tomatoes over each piece of salmon, covering the fish. Fold the parchment over to close the heart, and starting at top of heart shape, fold in both edges of parchment, overlapping folds as you move along the entire heart shape towards the bottom. When you reach the end tip, twist and fold under the packet. Packets should be tightly sealed.

Place packets on a baking sheet and bake for 15 minutes. When finished, serve on individual plates. With scissors, cut an "x" in top of each packet and peel back. Drizzle 2 tablespoons of *Balsamic Vinegar Reduction* within each open packet. What fun!

Serves 4

Eggplant Cacciatore

There's no need to sacrifice the mouth-watering satisfaction of a cacciatore dish just because you're avoiding meat and unhealthy fats. Here's a veggie version that's sure to satisfy that urge!

1 medium eggplant, cubed
3 tablespoons olive oil
1 large onion, chopped
1 red bell pepper, chopped
1 green bell pepper, chopped
½ pound mushrooms, chopped
3 garlic cloves, minced
1 (12 ounce) jar marinara sauce
1 (28 ounce) can whole tomatoes

1 (28 ounce) can diced tomatoes
1 cup pitted black olives, broken into pieces
¼ cup fresh chopped basil
¼ cup fresh chopped flat-leaf parsley
1 teaspoon dried oregano
2 tablespoons raw brown sugar
4 cups hot cooked whole wheat pasta (your choice)
Salt and pepper

Lightly salt the eggplant cubes and let sit for about 30 minutes to 'sweat.' Then rinse and pat dry with a paper towel. Heat 2 tablespoons oil in a medium saucepan over medium-high heat. Add onion, peppers, mushrooms, and garlic. Sauté until onions are caramelized and water is out of vegetables (about 20 minutes).

In a large skillet, heat another 1 tablespoon oil and sauté eggplant until water is removed and eggplant browns a little (about 10 minutes). Add marinara sauce, canned tomatoes, olives, spices, and brown sugar to saucepan with onions, peppers, and mushroom sauté. Mix well. Add browned eggplant and remainder of ingredients. Reduce heat and simmer mixture for 10-15 minutes. Salt and pepper to taste. Serve over whole wheat pasta.

Serves 4

Pasta Mushroom Sauce

Extracts of some mushrooms have been tested and shown to possibly help prevent breast cancer. In studies, the common white button mushroom had the strongest effect. Other mushrooms found to be helpful were portobello, cremini, and shitake, all found in your grocery aisle. So mix 'em up and enjoy!

3 tablespoons olive oil
1 small onion, finely chopped
3 cloves garlic, crushed
16 ounces fresh mushrooms, chopped (your choice, mix 'em up)
¼ cup red wine
2 cups nonfat chicken or vegetable broth

¼ cup chopped fresh flat-leaf parsley
1 tablespoon chopped fresh thyme
1 tablespoon chopped fresh sage
2 tablespoons cornstarch
2 tablespoons cold water
3 cups cooked whole wheat pasta
Salt and pepper

Enchilada Casserole

This is a great informal company meal. Everyone loves this dish, even the meat eaters! It's great because it can be put together a day ahead of time and then baked when your company arrives.

15 (6 inch) corn tortillas
1 (16 ounce) can fat-free refried beans
2 cups cooked brown rice
1 small bunch cilantro, chopped
1 small bunch flat-leaf parsley, chopped
2 bunches green onions, chopped
1 cup shredded cheese (part-skim mozzarella, veggie, or soy)

1 (28 ounce) can enchilada sauce
1 (15 ounce) can sweet corn, drained
1 (16 ounce) can pitted black olives, drained
Canola oil spray
Nonfat sour cream (optional)
Plain nonfat yogurt (optional)
Chopped avocado (optional)
Salsa (optional)

Preheat oven to 350 degrees F. Grease a 9" x 13" baking dish with olive oil spray. Place a tortilla in the palm of your hand and spread one heaping tablespoon of refried beans and add one tablespoon brown rice, ½ teaspoon chopped cilantro, ½ teaspoon chopped parsley, and 1 teaspoon chopped green onion. Roll up tortilla and place fold side down in the casserole pan. Repeat until the baking dish is full with one layer of rolled tortillas, placing each rolled tortilla side by side in pan. Don't be afraid to push the rolled tortillas together to squeeze in one more roll.

When the pan is full of rolled tortillas, spread cheese evenly on top. Pour enchilada sauce evenly over the top of the tortillas, then sprinkle with chopped pitted olives and corn. Cover with aluminum foil and bake in preheated oven for 45 minutes. Remove the foil for the last 15 minutes of baking. Serve with a large green salad and optional toppings, if desired. Enjoy!

Serves 8-10

In a large skillet, over medium heat, sauté the onions and garlic in the olive oil. Once the onions are soft, change the heat to medium-high and add the mushrooms. Cook until the water is out of the mushrooms, stirring constantly, about 5 minutes.

Add the red wine and stir well to release all of the brown bits from the bottom of the skillet. Add vegetable or chicken broth. Reduce heat and simmer for another 5 minutes. Add the parsley, thyme, and sage.

Combine the cornstarch and water until dissolved. Bring the sauce back up to a boil and whisk the cornstarch mixture into the sauce until the desired thickness is obtained. Reduce heat. Salt and pepper to taste. Serve hot over cooked whole wheat pasta.

Serves 3

Lasagna

Sometimes I just get a taste for Italian food. This is a nonfat, healthy version of an Italian classic. You won't miss the meat or the extra cheese, because there's plenty of flavor here, along with a great number of vitamins from the spinach and lycopene from the tomatoes.

1 pound whole wheat lasagna noodles
1 tablespoon olive oil
1 medium onion, diced
1 pound mushrooms, sliced
1 pound spinach, cleaned and cut up
64 ounces nonfat ricotta cheese
3 egg whites
½ cup chopped flat-leaf parsley
¼ cup chopped basil
3 cloves garlic, crushed
1 (26 ounce) jar nonfat or low-fat spaghetti sauce
6 ounces shredded cheese (part-skim mozzarella, veggie, or soy)
Salt and pepper
Canola oil spray

Preheat oven to 375 degrees F. Cook pasta al dente. Rinse, drain, and set aside.

Heat oil in a skillet and cook onion until caramelized (about 20 minutes). Add mushrooms and cook until much of the water from mushrooms is evaporated. Add spinach to skillet. Salt and pepper to taste and cook until all the water is evaporated. Set aside.

In a large bowl, combine ricotta cheese, egg whites, parsley, basil, and garlic. Salt and pepper to taste. Set aside.

Spray a 9" x 13" baking dish with canola oil. Pour 6 ounces of the spaghetti sauce on the bottom of the dish. Mix with 3 tablespoons water to cover the bottom of the pan.

Take ½ of the pasta and layer the bottom of the lasagna dish on top of the sauce. Spread the ricotta mixture carefully and evenly over the pasta. Spread the spinach mixture carefully and evenly over the ricotta. Sprinkle the cheese over the spinach. Take the remaining ½ of the pasta and layer it over the spinach. Take the remaining pasta sauce and pour it evenly over the top of the pasta. Cover with aluminum foil and bake in preheated oven for 45 minutes. Serve with a fresh, crisp salad and enjoy!

Serves 6-8

Mexican Polenta Casserole

This appetizing casserole is very low in fat and jam-packed with cancer-fighting ingredients: lycopene from the tomatoes, phytochemicals from the beans, peppers, parsley, and flavonoids from the onion. Don't forget the cancer-fighting properties of cumin!

2 tablespoons olive oil
1 large onion, diced
1 green pepper, diced
½ poblano pepper, diced
4 cloves garlic, crushed
1 (15 ounce) can black beans, rinsed and drained
1 tablespoon chili powder
2 tablespoons ground cumin
1 (14 ounce) can diced tomatoes, undrained

½ cup canned sweet corn, drained
¼ cup fresh chopped cilantro
¼ cup fresh chopped flat-leaf parsley
2 (16 ounce) tubes cooked polenta
1½ cups shredded cheese (part-skim mozzarella, veggie, or soy)
2 large tomatoes, sliced
1 small jalapeño pepper, seeded and diced finely (optional)
Olive oil spray

Preheat oven to 375 degrees F. In a large skillet, add 1 tablespoon of the olive oil, onion, peppers, and garlic. Sauté until the onions become translucent. Add black beans, chili powder, cumin, tomatoes, and corn. Add the jalapeño pepper (if desired). Bring to a boil and then reduce heat, cover, and simmer for 10-15 minutes. Add the parsley and the cilantro.

Spray a 9" x 13" baking dish with olive oil. Cut the polenta into ½ inch slices and press ½ of the slices firmly into the olive oil-sprayed baking dish. Pour the bean mixture over the polenta layer. Sprinkle half of the shredded cheese over the bean mixture. Place the remaining polenta slices over the cheese and beans. Sprinkle the remaining cheese over the polenta and place the sliced tomatoes on top.

Bake, uncovered, for 30 minutes. Allow to cool for 10-15 minutes before serving.

Serves 6-8

Moroccan Style Vegetables

Moroccan sauces are known for their combination of olives and lemons along with the medley of various other flavors. This sauce is sweet, hot, and savory all at the same time. Served over brown rice, it will satisfy your taste buds along with your nutritional needs!

2 tablespoons olive oil
2 onions, chopped
2 carrots, chopped
2 cups cauliflower, chopped
1 green pepper, chopped
2 cloves garlic, crushed
1 (14.5 ounce) can diced tomatoes, undrained
1 (15 ounce) can garbanzo beans (chickpeas), drained
¼ cup honey
⅓ cup raisins

12 green olives, chopped
¼ cup cilantro, chopped
Juice of one lemon
1 teaspoon cinnamon
1 tablespoon balsamic vinegar
1 teaspoon ground cumin
1 teaspoon paprika
3 bay leaves
3 cups cooked brown rice
Crushed red pepper flakes (optional)
Salt and pepper

Heat oil in a large skillet over medium heat. Cook onion, carrots, cauliflower, green pepper, and garlic in skillet until vegetables are al dente. Add the remaining ingredients (except rice, salt and pepper) and simmer for another 10 minutes or until vegetables are tender. Salt and pepper to taste. Add crushed red pepper flakes if so desired. Serve over cooked brown rice.

Serves 4-6

Poached Salmon with Rosemary

I don't eat a lot of salmon, as I eat primarily vegetarian, but this is a healthier way to cook the fish when I indulge. I'm calling it poached, but this method is a cross between poached and baked, since the salmon actually steams in the foil packet. It is cooked slowly in foil, so it is less likely to develop cancer-causing carcinogens that form during high-heat cooking.

4 (6 ounce) portions wild salmon
4 tablespoons white wine
½ teaspoon granulated garlic

4 small sprigs fresh rosemary (or dill)
Juice of 1 lemon
Salt and pepper

Dirty Rice

Enjoy a healthy version of this southern favorite. The brown rice and beans together make a complete protein, so adding some cooked chicken breast is optional. And beans are full of fiber!

2 tablespoons olive oil
1 small onion, chopped
½ poblano pepper, diced
½ red pepper, diced
1 cup carrots, diced
1 cup celery, diced
3 cloves garlic, minced
1 tablespoon cumin
1 tablespoon chili powder
1 tablespoon paprika
2 cups brown rice

2 large tomatoes, chopped
4 cups vegetable stock
1 bay leaf
1 (16 ounce) can kidney beans, rinsed and drained
½ cup chopped flat-leaf parsley
½ cup chopped cilantro
Salt and pepper
1 large chicken breast, cooked without skin and shredded (optional)
1 jalapeño pepper, minced (optional)

Heat the oil in a skillet over medium heat. Add the onion, peppers, carrot, and celery and sauté for 5 minutes. Add garlic and spices and cook until the vegetables are tender (5 minutes). Add all other ingredients (except for parsley and cilantro). Add shredded chicken breast and/or minced jalapeño if so desired. Simmer gently, uncovered, over low heat until the liquid is absorbed, about 30 minutes. Add parsley and cilantro. Salt and pepper to taste. Serve hot.

Serves 4-6

Preheat oven to 325 degrees F. Place each salmon portion in the center of a piece of aluminum foil large enough to fold over and totally cover the fish. Pour 1 tablespoon of white wine over each piece of salmon. Squeeze the lemon evenly over the 4 pieces of salmon, salt and pepper, and sprinkle granulated garlic over each piece. Place an individual sprig of rosemary on top of each piece of salmon.

Close the foil tightly around each piece. Place the foil packets onto a cookie sheet and place in preheated oven. Bake until done, about 10-15 minutes (time will vary depending on size of the salmon). Serve with *Avocado Sauce* or *Horseradish Sauce*. This can be served hot, or eaten cold the next day. It makes great picnic fare!

Serves 4

Pasta with Cauliflower, Broccoli, and Sun-Dried Tomatoes

Broccoli, cauliflower, and tomatoes have all been shown to have anti-cancer properties.

1 cup cauliflower, chopped
1 cup broccoli, chopped
3 tablespoons extra-virgin olive oil
1 onion, chopped
3 cloves garlic, minced
3 tablespoons pine nuts, roasted
2 tablespoons chopped fresh basil
1 tablespoon chopped fresh oregano

¼ cup sun-dried tomatoes in olive oil, drained and chopped
3 cups cooked whole wheat pasta
Salt and pepper
Extra-virgin olive oil for drizzling
2 tablespoons low-fat grated Parmesan cheese

Steam the broccoli and cauliflower to an el dente consistency. Remove from heat. In a large skillet, heat the olive oil. Add the garlic and onion and cook until the onion is caramelized. Add the pine nuts, broccoli, cauliflower, basil, oregano, and sun-dried tomatoes. Salt and pepper to taste. Add the cooked pasta and mix well. Drizzle with extra-virgin olive oil and sprinkle with Parmesan cheese.

Serves 3-4

Crusty Whitefish

All fish are not created equal. This dish calls for sablefish, also known as black cod. This fish is eco-friendly and one of the healthier whitefish, as it is high in omega 3s and its mercury content is moderate. If you cannot find sablefish, substitute wild caught Alaskan salmon. According to the Environmental Defense Fund (EDF) adults can eat 4+ servings per month of sablefish and children 2 (if no other contaminated fish is consumed). Wild caught Alaskan salmon is one of the healthier fish, and the EDF recommends 4+ servings per month of it for both adults and children.

4 (4 ounce) sablefish filets (from AK, CA, OR, WA, Canada)
5 tablespoons olive oil
Garlic powder

Salt and pepper
½ cup sliced almonds, rough chopped
1 cup Panko bread crumbs
Olive oil spray

Preheat oven to 350 degrees F. Place almonds on a cookie sheet and bake in oven for 5-10 minutes to toast. Watch carefully so they don't burn. Remove from oven. Set aside. Spray a cookie sheet with olive oil. Rub each piece of fish with 1 tablespoon olive oil on both sides. Place fish on olive oil-sprayed baking sheet. Sprinkle lightly with garlic powder. Salt and pepper each filet. In a small bowl, combine bread crumbs, nuts, and 1 tablespoon olive oil. Sprinkle crumb mixture evenly over each piece of fish, then spray with olive oil. Bake in preheated oven, about 20 minutes until fish is cooked and flakes easily with a fork. Drizzle each piece with lemon juice. Serve immediately.

Serves 4

Rice, Refried Beans, and Salad

So simple, so easy, and looks and tastes like a genuinely gourmet meal.

2 cups greens, finely sliced
1 cup halved cherry tomatoes
½ cup cucumber, chopped
¼ cup pitted black olives, chopped
3 tablespoons extra-virgin olive oil
2 tablespoons balsamic vinegar
Salt and pepper
3 corn tortillas

1 (15 ounce) can fat-free refried beans
¼ cup shredded cheese (part-skim mozzarella, veggie, or soy)
1 cup cooked brown rice
½ avocado, peeled and sliced
2 tablespoons chopped fresh cilantro
¼ cup salsa
¼ cup nonfat sour cream

In a medium bowl, toss greens, tomatoes, cucumber, and olives together. Dress with olive oil and vinegar. Set aside. Preheat oven to 400 degrees F. Cut tortillas in half. Place in a preheated oven for 10 minutes or until crisp. Remove from oven. Spread the refried beans out on two dinner plates. Spread the cheese evenly over the beans, and the rice evenly over the beans and cheese. Microwave for 1-2 minutes or until hot. Pour the salad evenly over the two plates. Garnish with sliced avocado, chopped cilantro, salsa, and sour cream. Place tortilla halves into side of beans for presentation.

Serves 2

Roasted Fennel Pasta

In research studies, fennel has been shown to reduce inflammation and to help prevent the occurrence of cancer. Fresh oregano has been shown to have more antioxidants than even blueberries!

2 fennel bulbs, stalks removed
½ cup olive oil
4 cloves garlic, crushed
1 large onion, diced
½ cup pitted black olives, chopped
2 large tomatoes, diced

3 tablespoons chopped fresh oregano
3 tablespoons chopped fresh basil
½ pound whole wheat pasta, cooked
¼ cup *Balsamic Vinegar Reduction*
Olive oil spray
Salt and pepper

Preheat oven to 400 degrees F. Spray a 9" x 13" baking dish with olive oil. Cut fennel into 1 inch pieces and toss with ¼ cup of olive oil until well coated. Sprinkle with salt and pepper and place in baking dish. Bake until fennel is caramelized on the edges, about 15-20 minutes. Stir a few times while roasting to prevent burning. In a large skillet, add the remaining ¼ cup olive oil, onion, and garlic. Cook until onions begin to caramelize (about 20 minutes) and add all other ingredients, including cooked fennel (except *Reduction*). Cook over medium heat, stirring until all ingredients are well mixed. Remove from heat, salt and pepper to taste, and serve immediately. Drizzle with *Balsamic Vinegar Reduction*.

Serves 4

Roasted Vegetables and Pasta

This recipe calls for a lot of veggies and a little pasta, which is a good ratio to abide by. Roasting vegetables brings out sweetness—remember, the antioxidants are in the veggies, not the pasta!

1 large red onion
1 pound portobello mushrooms
1 red bell pepper
1 green bell pepper
1 large zucchini
1 pound asparagus
2 large tomatoes
¼ cup extra-virgin olive oil
4 cloves garlic, crushed

8 ounces whole wheat pasta, cooked
2 tablespoons *Black Olive Tapenade*
2 tablespoons fresh oregano, chopped
2 tablespoons fresh basil, chopped
¼ cup low-fat grated Parmesan cheese
Salt and pepper
¼ cup *Balsamic Vinegar Reduction*
Olive oil spray

Preheat oven to 450 degrees F. Chop all vegetables into 1 inch pieces. Place all vegetables in a large bowl and coat with olive oil and chopped garlic. Spread your vegetables out onto 2 olive oil-sprayed baking sheets in single layers. Bake in the preheated oven for about 15-20 minutes. Check every 5 minutes and turn to brown on all sides. When the vegetables are roasted to your liking, toss with the pasta in a large bowl. Add the *Black Olive Tapenade*, oregano, and basil. Salt and pepper to taste. Add the Parmesan cheese and mix well. Drizzle with *Balsamic Vinegar Reduction* and serve hot.

Serves 4

Salmon Patties

I love this served with couscous and sautéed spinach, but topping it with *Hummus* or *Horseradish Sauce* really makes this dish.

16 ounces wild salmon, cooked
1 small onion, finely diced
1 stalk celery, chopped
¼ cup black olives, chopped
½ small red pepper, chopped
3 tablespoons chopped
fresh flat-leaf parsley

1 egg + 2 egg whites
¼ cup *Yogurt Cheese*
2 teaspoon prepared horseradish (optional)
1½ cups Panko bread crumbs
½ cup cornmeal
Olive oil spray
Salt and pepper

Place salmon into a large mixing bowl and flake with a fork. Mix in diced onion, celery, olives, red pepper, and parsley. Add eggs, *Yogurt Cheese*, and horseradish (if desired). Mix well. Add bread crumbs. Salt and pepper to taste. Shape into 4 patties. Dust patties in the cornmeal. Spray a large skillet with olive oil and sauté patties 2-3 minutes on each side.

Serves 4

Salmon Loaf

Here's a twist on the old meatloaf favorite. Think of it as satisfying the craving for comfort food, without all of the fat. This loaf can be served hot or cold (makes for a great picnic meal). Salmon is high in protein and omega-3 fatty acids and has long been known for its cancer prevention properties. Serve with either *Yogurt Dill Sauce, Avocado Dill Sauce,* or *Horseradish Sauce.* Recent research has shown that avocados help fight against prostate and oral cancer, and dill has shown anti-cancer properties.

2 pounds wild salmon, fresh, chopped finely
2 egg whites
¾ cup oatmeal (quick oats)
½ cup shredded cheese (part-skim mozzarella, veggie, or soy)
1 medium onion, finely diced
3 cloves garlic, minced
2 tablespoons chopped flat-leaf parsley
2 stalks celery, finely diced

2 tablespoons chopped fresh dill
Juice of one lemon
½ cup black olives, crushed
Zest of 1 lemon
½ teaspoon salt
½ teaspoon pepper
3-4 tomatoes, sliced, patted dry
Canola oil spray

Preheat oven to 350 degrees F. Mix all ingredients except tomatoes and canola oil spray. Transfer mixture into a 9" x 5" canola oil-sprayed loaf pan. Press down firmly. Slice tomatoes, seed, and arrange tomatoes on top of loaf. Sprinkle with salt and pepper. Bake in preheated oven for 1 hour or until done.

Serves 6-8

Vegetable Stir-Fry

Think outside the box and use a variety of vegetables. Brussels sprouts and cauliflower, for example, add an unusual variation to this classic stir-fry.

¼ pound Brussels sprouts, ends trimmed and halved
1 large carrot, chopped
1 bunch broccoli, cut up
2 tablespoons olive oil
2-3 cloves garlic, minced
1 large onion, chopped

¼ cauliflower, cut up
¼ pound green beans, trimmed, chopped
½ red bell pepper, sliced
½ green pepper, sliced
8 ounces mushrooms, sliced
2 tablespoons teriyaki sauce (low sodium)
2 cups cooked brown rice

Steam Brussels sprouts, carrot, and broccoli until half cooked. Set aside. Heat olive oil in a wok or large skillet. Add garlic and onion and cook until onions begin to caramelize (about 20 minutes). Add all other ingredients (except teriyaki sauce and rice). Stir well and cook on medium heat, stirring often until vegetables are tender and lightly browned (about 5-10 minutes). Add the teriyaki sauce and stir. Cook a few minutes more. Serve hot over brown rice or enjoy cold the next day!

Serves 4-6

Vegetable Brochettes

Why feel left out at summer cookouts because hamburgers, hot dogs, and ribs are no longer on your radar screen? These vegetable brochettes not only look great, as they couldn't be more colorful and inviting, they also taste great, so you don't have to feel excluded from the summer BBQ fun! One Memorial Day, I poured myself a glass of red wine, put some good music on, and hit the BBQ to begin grilling. I didn't feel slighted at all. Instead I felt blessed.

2 cups *Mushroom Rice*, or *Corn Rice*
1 large bunch broccoli, cleaned and cut into separate florets
1 large onion diced into 1 inch pieces
1 large cauliflower, washed and cut into separate large florets
2 large red peppers, cut in 1 inch pieces
2 large green peppers, cut in 1 inch pieces
1 pound cherry tomatoes

¼ red cabbage, cut in 1 inch pieces
2 ears corn, husked and cut in 1 inch pieces
16 large button mushrooms
4 large carrots, cleaned, ends trimmed, and cut in 1 inch pieces
2 large summer squash, cut in 1 inch pieces
Salt and pepper
Granulated garlic
Olive oil spray

Spicy Red Beans and Lentils

Lentils are a miracle food. High in protein, when combined with brown rice they supply your body with a complete protein. They are high in fiber and can help lower your cholesterol. Lentils are versatile, inexpensive, high in Vitamin B, and studies have shown that they help prevent cancer. What more could you ask them to do?

2 tablespoons olive oil
4 cloves garlic, minced
1 red bell pepper, diced
2 (15 ounce) cans red beans, drained
2 cups vegetable broth
1 teaspoon ground cumin
1 teaspoon ground coriander
½ teaspoon chili powder

1 (28 ounce) can whole tomatoes
1 cup plain nonfat yogurt
1 cup lentils, rinsed (preferably red)
1 tablespoon raw brown sugar
¼ cup chopped flat-leaf parsley
¼ cup chopped cilantro
Salt and pepper
1 small jalapeño, chopped finely (optional)

In a large pot, add olive oil, garlic, and red pepper. Stirring often, cook until peppers are soft. Add all other ingredients, except yogurt, and bring to a boil. Reduce heat to a simmer, cover, and cook until lentils are tender, about 45 minutes. Salt and pepper to taste. Stir in yogurt and serve over brown rice.

Serves 4-6

Precook the broccoli, peppers, cabbage, carrots, and squash to an al dente state. You do this step first, so you don't burn the vegetables on the grill. I have a microwave steamer that I precook each variety of vegetable in. Once vegetables have cooled from being precooked, arrange vegetables on 8 skewers, alternating types until all vegetables are used.

Spray brochettes with olive oil, making sure you turn the skewers to get all sides of vegetables. Sprinkle each brochette with salt, pepper, and granulated garlic. Grill on well-oiled, preheated grill until desired doneness is obtained. Serve 2 skewers over ½ cup of rice.

Note: If any vegetables are left over, use in a stir fry!

Serves 4

Marinated Tomatoes

I like to vary my types to achieve a variety of tastes in this dish. Mix it up with whatever is in season, and don't be afraid to try something new.

1 pound tomatoes, chopped
1 large clove garlic, crushed
¼ cup chopped fresh basil
¼ cup chopped fresh cilantro
2 tablespoons balsamic vinegar
2 tablespoons extra-virgin olive oil
Salt and pepper

Mix all ingredients together and let the mixture sit in the refrigerator for an hour before serving, to allow the flavors to meld together. Stir again before serving. Salt and pepper to taste.

Spinach, Mustard Greens, and Pesto Pasta

Although traditionally made with basil, pesto can really be made with any greens. Adding mustard greens to this favorite bumps up the nutritional level considerably. Mustard green leaves are loaded with vitamins, minerals, and dietary fiber. As a matter of fact, they are known to have high amounts of 16 different vitamins and minerals! Mustard greens are a member of the cabbage (Brassica) family, which has been shown to contain the cancer-fighting phytonutrient glucosinolate.

5 cloves garlic
½ cup walnuts
¼ cup low-fat grated Parmesan cheese
¼ cup extra-virgin olive oil
Juice of one lemon

1 cup (packed) fresh mustard greens, washed and dried
1 cup (packed) fresh spinach, cleaned
Salt and pepper
10 ounces whole wheat pasta, uncooked

Process garlic, walnuts, Parmesan cheese, oil, and lemon juice in a food processor until blended. Add mustard greens and spinach, bit by bit, until all greens are processed. Salt and pepper to taste. Boil pasta according to package directions and then drain. In a large bowl, combine the pesto and pasta. Serve hot. Top with *Marinated Tomatoes*.

Serves 3-4

Turkey Meatloaf

Nothing beats meatloaf as comfort food, but we want to avoid eating red meat. I don't eat this often because of the meat (even though it's turkey or chicken) and the ketchup (even though it's organic). Once or twice a year, I make this healthier version to satisfy a craving. While it is healthier than the traditional ground beef meatloaf, it still is not a cancer fighter. That being said, you probably won't even be able to tell the difference between it and the traditional!

2 pounds ground, 99% fat-free white meat turkey or chicken
½ cup organic ketchup (no high-fructose corn syrup and limited sugar)
½ cup warm water
2 egg whites
1¼ cups oatmeal (quick oats)
1 tablespoon Worcestershire sauce (organic, no high-fructose corn syrup)

2 tablespoons dehydrated onions
1 teaspoon celery salt
1 teaspoon garlic powder
½ teaspoon cracked black pepper
½ teaspoon paprika
½ teaspoon celery seed
3-4 tomatoes, sliced
Canola oil spray

Preheat oven to 350 degrees F. Mix all ingredients except tomatoes thoroughly. Put into a 9" x 5" canola oil-sprayed loaf pan. Press down firmly. Slice tomatoes and drain them on a paper towel. Arrange tomatoes on top of meatloaf. Bake in preheated oven for 1 hour or until done.

Serves 6-8

Stuffed Peppers

Sweet bell peppers are excellent sources of both Vitamin A and Vitamin C, two very powerful antioxidants. These peppers are stuffed with a wild rice mixture and vegetables instead of meat, which makes them high in fiber and vitamins.

6 large sweet peppers: red, green, or yellow
3 tablespoons olive oil
1 large onion, diced
1 large carrot, diced
2 large celery ribs, diced
8 ounces button mushrooms, sliced
3 garlic cloves, crushed
2 large tomatoes, seeded and chopped
2 tablespoons fresh chopped basil leaves
1 tablespoon fresh chopped oregano

¼ cup fresh chopped flat-leaf parsley
Salt and pepper
3 cups cooked wild rice
1 cup shredded cheese (part-skim mozzarella, veggie, or soy)
¼ cup low-fat grated Parmesan cheese
Olive oil spray

Southern Style Rice and Beans

Beans are so good for you. That's any and all beans, canned, dried, whatever. Beans are great protein and fiber, and also provide essential minerals. This is an easy 1-pan meal that is sure to please. The poblano pepper gives it just the right amount of kick. Serve as a main dish with a salad, or serve as a side.

1 tablespoon extra-virgin olive oil
1 small onion, diced
1 poblano pepper, diced (Substitute a green bell pepper for mild flavor)
1 red pepper, seeded and diced
1 stalk celery, diced
2 cloves garlic, minced
1 carrot, diced
½ pound mushrooms, sliced

1 tablespoon paprika
1 tablespoon chopped fresh oregano
1 tablespoon chopped fresh thyme
1 (15 ounce) can black beans, drained
1½ cups vegetable broth
1 (14 ounce) can diced tomatoes
2 cups brown rice, uncooked
Salt and pepper
Crushed red pepper flakes (optional)

Heat the oil in a large skillet and add the onions, peppers, celery, garlic, carrot, and mushrooms. Cook for about 5 minutes. The vegetables will be semi-cooked. Add the remaining ingredients and mix well. Bring to a boil, reduce heat to simmer, and cover. Continue cooking until rice is cooked, about 40 minutes. Salt and pepper to taste. Add dried pepper flakes if desired.

Serves 3-4

Preheat oven to 350 degrees F. Cut tops off peppers and remove seeds. Par-cook the peppers by placing them in a large baking dish with 1 inch of water. Cover the pan and place in the preheated oven for 15 minutes. Remove from the oven, remove the peppers, dry the dish, spray it with olive oil, and set aside.

In a large skillet, add the olive oil, onions, carrots, celery, mushrooms, and garlic. Cook until onions are translucent, the carrots are soft, and the water has cooked out of the mushrooms. Add the tomatoes, basil, oregano, and parsley. Salt and pepper to taste. Remove from heat.

In a large bowl, combine the rice and the cooked vegetable mixture, and stir until well mixed. Stir in the cheese. Spoon into the par-cooked peppers. Sprinkle with Parmesan cheese. Cover the pan with foil and bake 30 minutes. Remove the foil and continue to bake for another 10 minutes. Serve with your favorite low-fat pasta sauce.

Serves 3-4

Roasted Veggie Fajitas

This is a fun recipe to entertain with. People love to design their own fajita with personal toppings, and these are loaded with lots of cancer-fighting veggies and garlic. Even the cumin has cancer-fighting properties!

1 red bell pepper, cut in strips
1 green bell pepper, cut in strips
1 yellow bell pepper, cut in strips
1 large onion, diced
1 large tomato, diced
1 yellow summer squash or
1 zucchini, diced
½ pound button mushrooms, sliced
3 tablespoons olive oil
2 large cloves garlic, minced
1 teaspoon cumin

1 teaspoon chili powder
Salt and pepper
Juice of 1 lime
4 whole wheat 10 inch tortillas
3 cups cooked brown rice
Shredded spinach (optional)
Nonfat sour cream (optional)
Sliced avocado (optional)
Salsa (optional)
Fresh chopped cilantro (optional)

Veggie Burritos

These burritos are chock full of antioxidant-loaded veggies and fresh herbs, low-fat, and high fiber. Bell peppers, onions, carrots, garlic, oregano, and basil have all been found to have cancer-fighting properties.

3 tablespoons olive oil
1 large onion, chopped
2 tablespoons garlic, minced
2 zucchini, chopped
1 red bell pepper, cut in strips
1 green bell pepper, cut in strips
1 large tomato, diced
1 cup carrots, sliced thinly
8 ounces fresh button mushrooms, sliced
1 cup canned sweet corn, drained
1 tablespoon chopped fresh oregano

1 tablespoon chopped fresh basil
1 tablespoon chili powder
½ teaspoon cumin
Salt and pepper
Canola oil spray
4 whole wheat 10 inch tortillas
Nonfat sour cream (optional)
Sliced avocado (optional)
Chopped greens (optional)
Chopped tomatoes (optional)
Salsa (optional)

In a large skillet, over medium heat, add the oil, onion, and garlic. Cook until the onion begins to become translucent. Add all of the remaining ingredients (except the oregano, basil, chili powder, cumin, and salt and pepper). Stir well, reduce heat, and continue to cook until the vegetables are tender. Add the oregano, basil, chili powder, and cumin. Mix well and cook for another 5 minutes, stirring often. Salt and pepper to taste. Warm the tortilla either in the microwave or oven. Spoon ½ cup of vegetable mixture onto each tortilla, fold over edges, and roll up. Serve immediately with optional toppings.

Serves 4

Preheat oven to 400 degrees F. Place all vegetables in a large bowl and coat with olive oil, crushed garlic, cumin, chili powder, and salt and pepper. Spread coated vegetables onto a large cookie sheet evenly.

Place vegetables into the preheated oven until tender, stirring occasionally (about 15-20 minutes). Warm the tortillas and prepare the toppings.

Once the vegetables are cooked to the desired tenderness, squeeze the lime over the vegetables and serve over brown rice and with optional toppings. Serve with warm tortillas.

Serves 4

Spinach and Mushroom Quesadillas

If you love Mexican food, especially those fat-filled cheese quesadillas—surprise! You don't have to give up their flavor and texture. Try this low-fat recipe that's chock full of ingredients with cancer-fighting antioxidants and phytochemicals.

2 tablespoons extra-virgin olive oil
1 small onion, chopped
½ pound fresh mushrooms, sliced
1 pound cleaned fresh spinach, chopped
½ cup shredded cheese (part-skim mozzarella, veggie, or soy)

4 (6 inch) whole wheat tortillas
Salt and pepper
Salsa (optional)
Sliced avocado (optional)
Plain nonfat yogurt (optional)

Heat olive oil in a sauté pan and add onion. Sauté until translucent. Add mushrooms and cook until tender (4-5 minutes). Add spinach and cook until spinach is cooked down in volume. Salt and pepper to taste. Set aside. Heat tortillas on top of a grill or in a 350 degrees F oven until warm and toasted on both sides. Place 2 tortillas side by side. Place ¼ cup of the shredded cheese evenly over the two tortillas. Divide the spinach mixture atop the same 2 tortillas with the cheese. Spread the spinach mixture almost to the ends of the tortillas. Place the remaining cheese evenly atop the spinach mixture. Place the 2 remaining toasted plain tortillas atop the tortillas with the spinach and cheese on them. Press down to flatten the tortilla "sandwich" as much as possible. Toast for 2 minutes more on each side, either on the grill or in the oven, just enough to melt the cheese and reheat the spinach mixture. Serve with optional toppings.

Serves 2-3

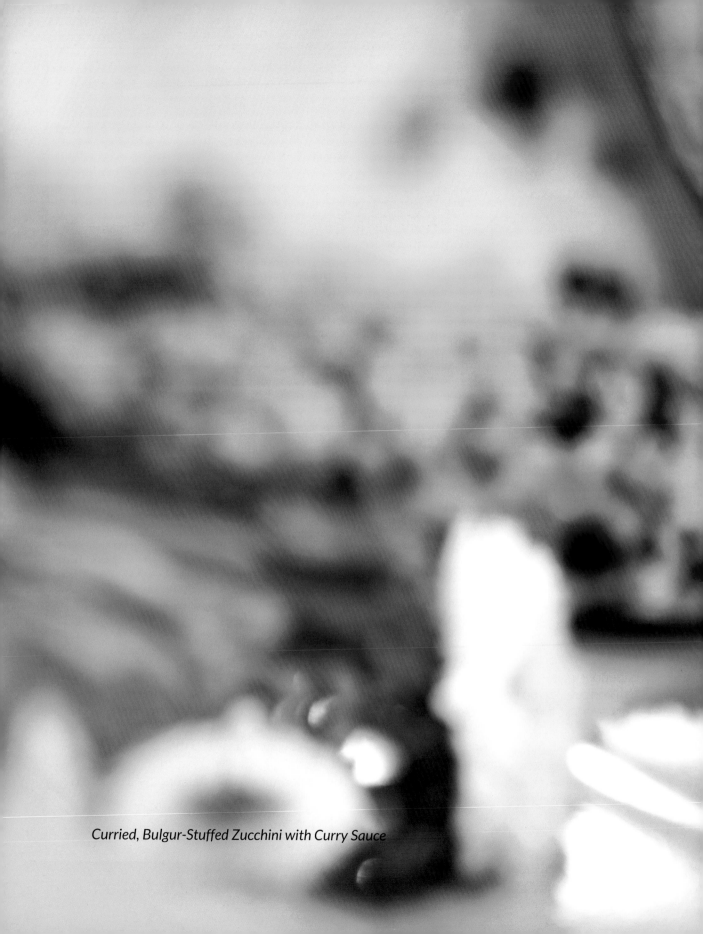

Curried, Bulgur-Stuffed Zucchini with Curry Sauce

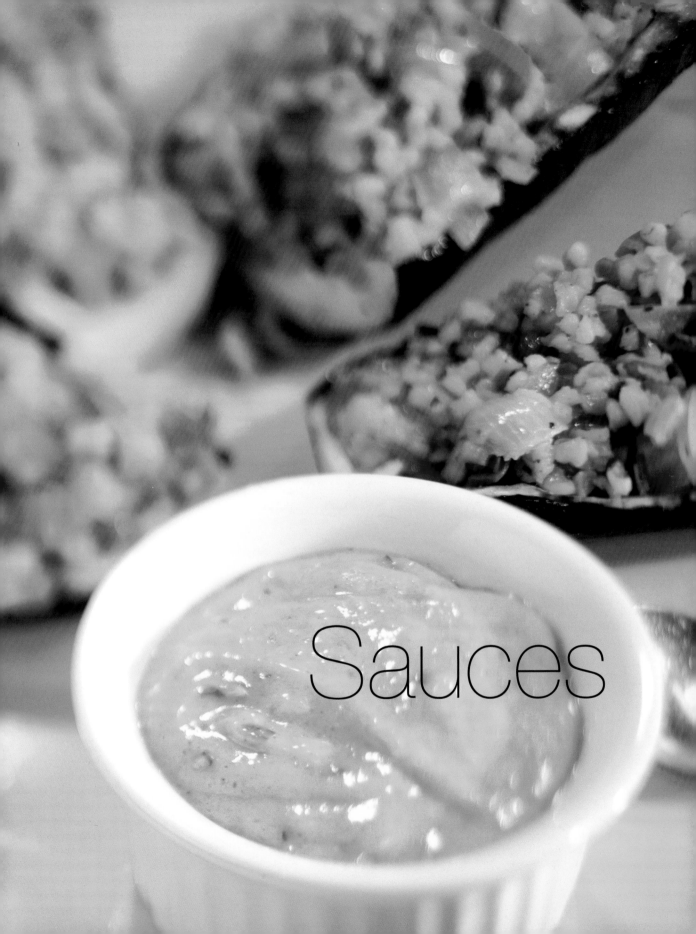

Sauces

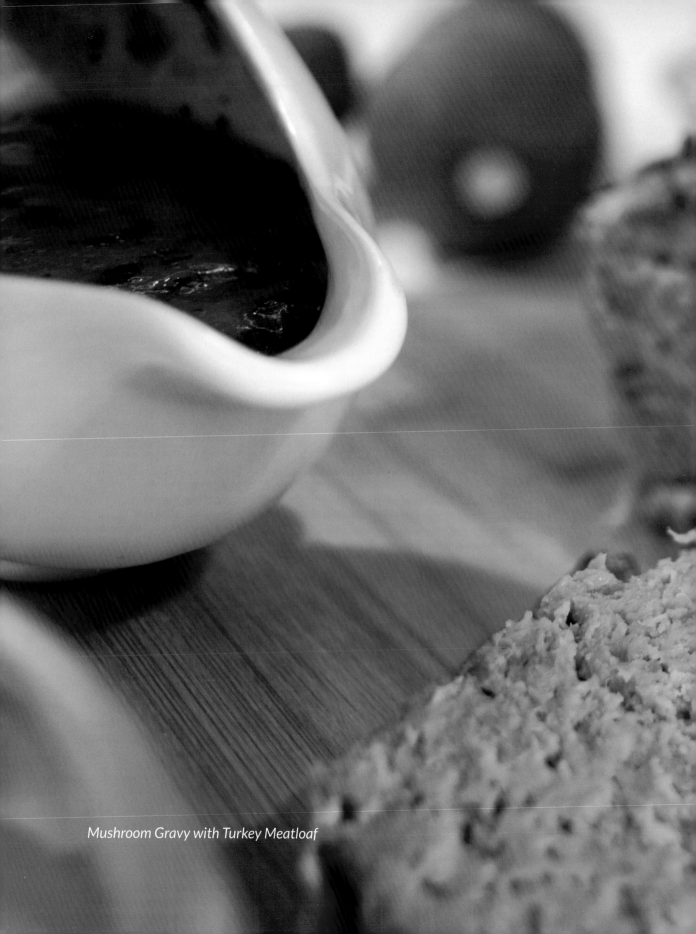

Mushroom Gravy with Turkey Meatloaf

Ah, sauces! They can add a gourmet touch to almost any meal. Sauces are truly a way of accessorizing your cooking, taking a "blah" meal to an "ahh!" meal.

The problem with most sauces is that they begin or end with butter, and that's a no-no when we want to avoid unhealthy fats in our diets. The wonderful surprise I've found is that you don't have to sacrifice the delectable treat of a saucy meal to make it healthy! These sauces do not contain butter, yet they don't sacrifice taste at all. As a matter of fact, I'd be surprised if anybody could tell the difference between these and fat-laden sauces.

It goes to show that made properly, even sauces can be made healthfully!

Homemade Apple Sauce

Your mother or grandmother was probably correct when she told you, "An apple a day keeps the doctor away." A compound in apples may prove to be a natural fighter against colon cancer.

6 large apples
2 teaspoons honey
½ cup raisins

1 teaspoon cinnamon
½ teaspoon nutmeg
½ cup orange juice

Preheat oven to 350 degrees F. Peel, core, and slice the apples, then add honey, raisins, cinnamon, and nutmeg. Toss together until mixed well. Spread the mixture across the bottom of a 9" x 13" baking dish. Pour the orange juice into the bottom of the baking dish. Cover with aluminum foil and cook in preheated oven for 45 minutes or until apples are soft. Remove foil and cook for another 10 minutes. Allow to cool, then blend in a food processor until semi-smooth. Refrigerate. Serve cold.

Note: You can also blend half of the mixture and serve on top of remainder of apple mixture warm as a dessert.

Balsamic Vinegar Reduction

This sauce is easy to make, and it really adds the finishing touch to a dish. In essence, all you do is take ordinary balsamic vinegar, and reduce it by 50%. Here are a couple of ways to make it. If you are an inexperienced cook, I would recommend Cooking Method #2, since balsamic vinegar is fairly easy to scorch if not whisked constantly, and scorched vinegar will render the reduction unusable. Cooking Method #2 is pretty much fool-proof.

2 cups balsamic vinegar

Cooking Method #1

Pour balsamic vinegar into a saucepan. Place pan on a high heat and whisk briskly and constantly to prevent scorching. When vinegar is reduced by 50% in volume and thickens, remove from heat immediately (watch the vinegar closely; when the vinegar begins to thicken, it will happen quickly). Pour into a different container to avoid vinegar continuing to cook. Additional spices of your choice such as thyme or garlic can also be added at this time.

Cooking Method #2

Place vinegar in the top of a double boiler. Cook slowly, stirring often until liquid is reduced by 50% (watch the vinegar closely; when the vinegar begins to thicken, it will happen quickly). Remove from stove and pour into a different container to avoid vinegar continuing to cook. Additional spices of your choice such as thyme or garlic can also be added at this time.

Black Bean Sauce

I can't say enough about beans. They are a big miracle in a tiny little package. They are high in protein and fiber, low in fat, and loaded with vitamins and minerals.

1 tablespoon canola oil
1 small onion, chopped finely
2 cloves garlic, minced
8 ounces black beans, drained and rinsed
8 ounces organic chili beans, drained and rinsed

1 cup chicken or vegetable stock
2 medium tomatoes, diced
¼ cup chopped cilantro
¼ cup chopped flat-leaf parsley
1 teaspoon cumin
½ teaspoon chili powder (optional)
Salt and pepper

In a medium skillet, heat the oil, onions, and garlic. Sauté until the onions are translucent. Place beans and stock in a large sauce pan and bring to a boil. Add the sautéed onions and garlic. Add the tomatoes. Reduce heat and simmer, stirring often until all ingredients are soft and well mixed (about 10 minutes). Add the parsley and cilantro. Season with cumin. Add chili powder if desired. Salt and pepper to taste. With a hand blender or potato masher, blend slightly but not thoroughly. Sauce should be chunky. Serve hot over *Journey Cakes* or over brown rice or any whole grain.

Cucumber Yogurt Dip

This is a versatile dip that can be used for dipping raw vegetables or chips. You can even put it on a sandwich as a tasty substitute for mayonnaise or use it as a salad dressing.

1 cup *Yogurt Cheese*
1 large cucumber, seeded and diced finely
1 cup nonfat sour cream
Juice of one lemon
Zest of one lemon

1 tablespoon raw brown sugar
2 tablespoons chopped flat-leaf parsley
2 cloves garlic, minced
2 tablespoons chopped fresh dill
Salt and pepper

Blot the cucumber with a clean kitchen towel to dry it as much as possible. Combine all ingredients in a large bowl and stir until well blended. Cover and place in the refrigerator and allow to chill for at least 4 hours. Serve chilled.

Curry Sauce

Curry is considered by some to be the miracle spice, as it is being avidly studied for its cancer-fighting properties. This creamy sauce can be served over rice, vegetables, or fish.

2 tablespoons canola oil
1 tablespoon cornstarch
½ cup nonfat milk
½ cup vegetable stock or
fat-free chicken stock
¼ cup nonfat sour cream

1 tablespoon curry powder
1 tablespoon finely chopped basil
1 tablespoon finely chopped
flat-leaf parsley
Salt and pepper

In a medium saucepan, whisk together oil and cornstarch over a medium heat. Whisk in the milk and vegetable stock, slowly bringing to a boil, until all lumps dissolve and mixture is thick. Add sour cream, curry, basil, and parsley. Whisk together until thoroughly blended. Salt and pepper to taste. Serve hot.

Garlic Yogurt Dip

I like to eat this dip with marinated artichokes, but it can be paired with pita chips or used as a dressing.

1 cup *Yogurt Cheese*
4 cloves garlic, minced
1 cup nonfat sour cream
1 tablespoon raw brown sugar

Juice of one lemon
Zest of one lemon
Salt and pepper

Combine all ingredients in a large bowl and whisk until well blended. Cover and place in the refrigerator and allow to chill for at least 4 hours. Serve chilled.

Horseradish Sauce

Horseradish is loaded with glucosinolates, the same compounds in broccoli that have shown to increase human resistance to cancer. Spoon some of this sauce over a roasted veggie sandwich, a piece of fish, a salmon burger, or even some fresh cooked beets.

1 tablespoon prepared horseradish
½ cup nonfat sour cream or *Yogurt Cheese*
1 tablespoon Worcestershire sauce
(organic, no high-fructose corn syrup)
¼ teaspoon raw brown sugar

¼ cup faux buttermilk (¼ cup nonfat milk
and ½ teaspoon lemon juice)
2 tablespoons chopped flat-leaf parsley
1 tablespoon chopped chives
Salt and pepper

Whisk all ingredients together until smooth. Serve chilled.

Hummus Sauce

This sauce is great over fish or vegetables. It's high in protein and high in fiber.

1 (16 ounce) can garbanzo beans (chickpeas), include ½ of liquid
Juice of one lemon
1 tablespoon tahini
2 cloves garlic, minced

1 tablespoon olive oil
¼ cup chopped cilantro
¼ cup white wine or water
Salt and pepper

Place all ingredients in a food processor and blend until smooth.

Yogurt Dill Sauce

This sauce tastes great on a *Salmon Burger* or drizzled over *Salmon Loaf*. It can also be used for dipping.

1 cup plain nonfat yogurt
3 tablespoons chopped fresh dill
2 large garlic cloves, minced

Juice of 1 fresh lemon
1 teaspoon raw brown sugar
Salt and pepper to taste

Place all ingredients in a food processor and blend until smooth.

Fresh Fruit Dessert Compote

This dessert can be served all year round, hot or cold. Fruits and berries contain potent antioxidants.

½ cup apple juice
¼ cup honey
1 teaspoon vanilla
Juice of one lemon
Zest of one lemon
2 apples, cored and sliced
2 peaches, pitted and sliced

1 pear, cored and sliced
1 cup sliced strawberries
1 cup blueberries
1 cup seedless red grapes
1 tablespoon cornstarch
1 tablespoon cold water

In a large saucepan, combine the apple juice, honey, vanilla, lemon juice, and zest. Mix well. Add the apples, peaches, and pear and bring to a boil. Reduce heat and continue cooking for 10 minutes. Add strawberries, blueberries, and grapes and cook for another 10 minutes. Change heat to medium high and bring to a low boil. Combine cornstarch and cold water in a cup and mix well until cornstarch dissolves. Add to the fruit. Cook for another minute, stirring constantly. Compote should thicken quickly. Remove from heat. Serve warm or chill to serve cold. Store covered in the refrigerator.

Mojo Sauce

Mojo is a Cuban sauce that's generally used on meats, but it's equally good on fish or veggies. It also makes a great marinade. Try it on a veggie sandwich or panini. Bueno!

6 medium garlic cloves, minced
1 teaspoon lime zest
3 tablespoons fresh lime juice
1 teaspoon orange zest
3 tablespoons fresh orange juice
½ teaspoon ground cumin

½ teaspoon salt
1 teaspoon honey
1 tablespoon chopped cilantro
½ cup extra-virgin olive oil
Salt and pepper

Put all ingredients (except oil and salt and pepper) in a blender. Pulse until finely chopped. While the blender is still running, add the oil slowly until it's emulsified. Salt and pepper to taste. Keep refrigerated.

Mushroom Gravy

No meat drippings needed for a tasty gravy that satisfies over a mound of *Roasted Garlic Mashed Potatoes*.

2 tablespoons olive oil
1 large clove garlic, minced
1 pound mushrooms, sliced
2 cups vegetable broth
1 teaspoon Kitchen Bouquet

1 teaspoon cornstarch, completely dissolved in ¼ cup of cold water
1 tablespoon sherry
¼ cup chopped flat-leaf parsley
Salt and pepper

Sauté mushrooms and garlic until mushrooms are cooked and water evaporates. Add broth and bring to a boil. Add cornstarch mixture, whisking constantly until gravy is desired consistency (if it gets too thick, add a little more broth). Stir in Kitchen Bouquet, sherry, and parsley. Salt and pepper to taste. Serve immediately.

Pesto

Pesto is classic, simple, and versatile. Combine basil, spinach, and garlic and you can't go wrong.

1 cup basil leaves, well packed
1 cup spinach or kale leaves, well packed
3 cloves garlic, crushed
¼ cup walnuts
¼ cup pistachio nuts, shelled

¼ cup low-fat grated Parmesan cheese
½-cup extra-virgin olive oil (use more or less to obtain desired consistency)
Salt and pepper

Place all ingredients (except salt and pepper) in a food processor or blender and process until well combined. Salt and pepper to taste. Serve on a pizza or over fish, veggies, pasta, or baguette slices.

Onion Butter

This is an old fashioned favorite and a healthy topping for your toast, veggies, or fish. Onion butter makes a great dipping sauce and couldn't be simpler to prepare. Cooking the onions down slowly will make a creamy, excellent replacement for butter thats totally worth the wait.

5 pounds onions (your choice of variety)
Water

6 cloves garlic (optional)
Salt and pepper

Peel and roughly chop the onions. Place the onions (and garlic if desired) in a large pot and cover with water. Bring to a boil then reduce heat to a simmer. Allow the onions to cook for at least 8 hours. Onions will be brown and soft. Stir occasionally throughout the cooking process and keep adding more water when necessary to avoid burning. When onions are soft, set the heat to high just long enough to boil out all of the remaining water. Stir constantly while the heat is on high. With an electric hand blender, blend the onions until smooth. Salt and pepper to taste. The onion butter will store in your refrigerator for at least a week in a covered container, if it doesn't get eaten up first!

Cilantro Sauce

Cilantro is a little herb with big possibilities. It has been shown to improve both memory and digestion.

1 small onion, chopped
¼ cup extra-virgin olive oil + 1 tablespoon
1 cup cilantro, packed
2 garlic cloves, minced

Juice of 1 lime
¼ teaspoon salt
¼ teaspoon cracked black pepper

In a small skillet, sauté the onion in 1 tablespoon olive oil until onion is soft and has some color. Place all ingredients, including onion, into a food processor and pulse until well combined.

Caramelized Onions with Balsamic Vinegar

What a tasty treat this is! Caramelized onions can be served over potatoes, vegetables, or fish. Studies have shown that onions probably decrease the risk of stomach cancer.

2 large onions, thinly sliced
2 tablespoons olive oil

2 tablespoons balsamic vinegar

In a large skillet, heat the oil and then add the onions. Stir on high heat for 1 minute and then reduce heat to low. Cook slowly, stirring occasionally, until onions are soft and brown. Be careful not to burn them. Be patient. Caramelizing the onions can take 30-45 minutes. When onions are dark golden brown, turn heat to medium-high, add vinegar, and stir. Remove from heat. Serve immediately or store in the refrigerator until ready to use. These will keep in the refrigerator for up to 1 week.

Pineapple Salsa

Pineapple contains a natural substance called bromelain, which in laboratory research has been shown to reduce inflammation, metastasis, and tumor growth, leading to an increase in survival rates.

1 small pineapple, skin and core removed
1 large red onion, quartered
1 red bell pepper, diced
¼ cup cilantro, chopped

Juice of one lime
Zest of one lime
Salt and pepper

Cut the pineapple into slices and cook, along with onion, on a medium-hot, oiled grill until slightly caramelized. Allow to cool. Chop into ¼ inch pieces and add the remaining ingredients. Mix well.

Portobello Relish

This relish can be served hot or cold, over vegetables or fish, or it can stand on it's own as a side dish.

4 large portobello mushrooms
1 red onion, diced finely
1 red bell pepper, seeded and diced
1 green bell pepper, seeded and diced
4 cloves garlic, minced
2 tablespoons olive oil

2 tablespoons balsamic vinegar
½ teaspoon chopped fresh rosemary
½ teaspoon fresh thyme
2 tablespoons capers
Salt and pepper
Olive oil spray

Spray the mushrooms with the olive oil spray. Place on a hot grill or griddle and cook until soft. Remove from heat and allow to cool, then chop into small pieces. In a large skillet, heat the olive oil over a medium heat. Add the onions, peppers, and garlic and cook until soft. Remove from heat. In a large bowl, combine the mushrooms and pepper mixture. Mix well. Add the olive oil, balsamic vinegar, rosemary, thyme, and capers. Salt and pepper to taste. Chill for at least 4 hours before serving.

Avocado Dill Sauce

This sauce tastes great on a salmon burger or drizzled over a salmon loaf. You can use it for dipping, too. Both avocados and dill have been shown in studies to have cancer fighting properties. Here's another instance of *what tastes good can be good for you*!

1 ripe avocado, mashed
Juice of 1 lemon
2 tablespoons chopped fresh dill

1 teaspoon raw brown sugar
2 tablespoons white wine
Salt and pepper

Place all ingredients in a food processor and blend until smooth. Serve chilled.

Creole Sauce

Creole sauce is a versatile dish that can be served over fish, grains, or eggs. It's bound to perk up a meal!

2 tablespoons olive oil
4 ounces fresh mushrooms, sliced
2 stalks celery, diced
½ green pepper, cut in 1 inch squares
1 small onion, chopped
1 large garlic clove, minced

6 ounce can tomato paste
8 ounces vegetable broth
1 teaspoon fresh chopped oregano
1 teaspoon fresh thyme
1 tablespoon fresh chopped basil
Salt and pepper

In a small skillet, over medium-high heat, sauté the mushrooms with 1 tablespoon olive oil until brown. Set aside. In a medium skillet, over medium-high heat, sauté celery, green pepper, onion, and garlic in olive oil for about two or three minutes. Do not overcook. The vegetables should remain crisp-tender. Add tomato paste and broth. Add mushrooms, oregano, thyme, and basil. Cover and simmer gently for about 10 minutes, stirring occasionally to prevent burning. Salt and pepper to taste. Serve over whole wheat pasta, brown rice, or bulgar.

Yogurt Cheese

1 quart plain nonfat yogurt

Cut a piece of cheesecloth so that the length is about four times the width of the strainer or colander you are using. Line the strainer or colander with two layers of the cheesecloth. Place the strainer over a large bowl. Empty the yogurt container into the strainer. Pull the ends of the cheesecloth up over the yogurt to cover it.

Place a plate on top of the cheesecloth that is slightly smaller in diameter than the top of the strainer or colander. You want the plate to sit directly on top of the cheesecloth covering the yogurt without touching the rim of the strainer or colander. Place something heavy on top of the plate to weight it down. (I use a rock from my garden covered in foil, but you could use a can of soup, a bag of beans, anything heavy.)

Put into the refrigerator and allow to sit for anywhere from 1 hour to 24 hours. The longer you leave it sit, the more whey will drain out of it and the thicker it will become. If you leave it for an hour or two, it will become the consistency of sour cream. If you leave it for 24 hours, it will become the consistency of cream cheese. If you leave it for the longer period of time, you will probably need to occasionally empty the whey out of the bowl (depending on the size of the bowl) so the strainer doesn't sit in the liquid whey.

After the whey leaks out of the yogurt into the bowl, take off the weight and the plate and gently squeeze any liquid that is left out of the yogurt. Discard the liquid. Place the yogurt into an airtight container and store in the refrigerator until used.

Note: You can also use coffee filters in a small strainer if you don't have any cheesecloth.

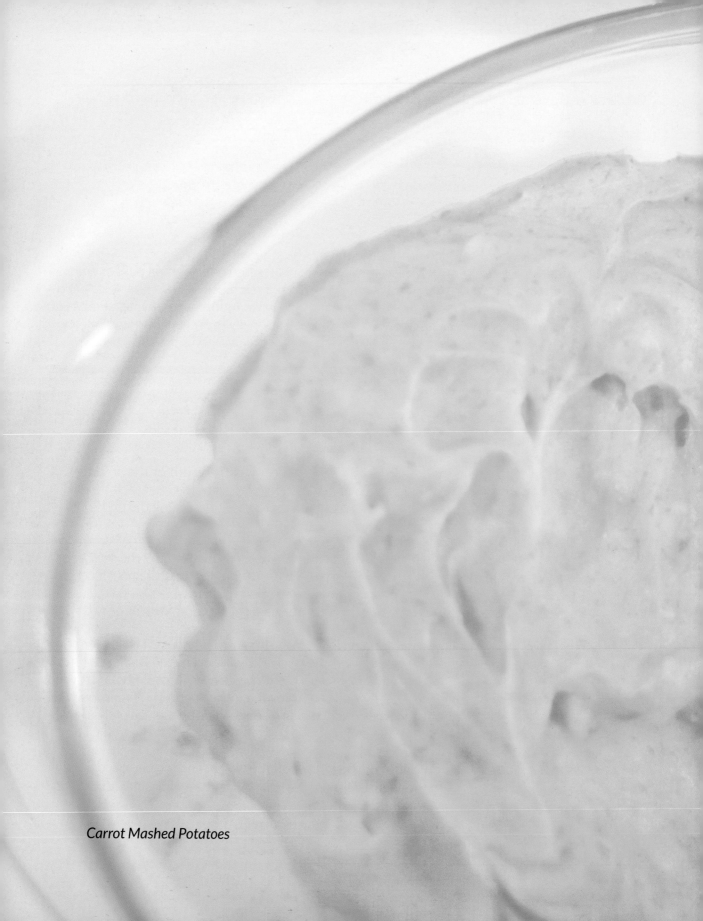

Carrot Mashed Potatoes

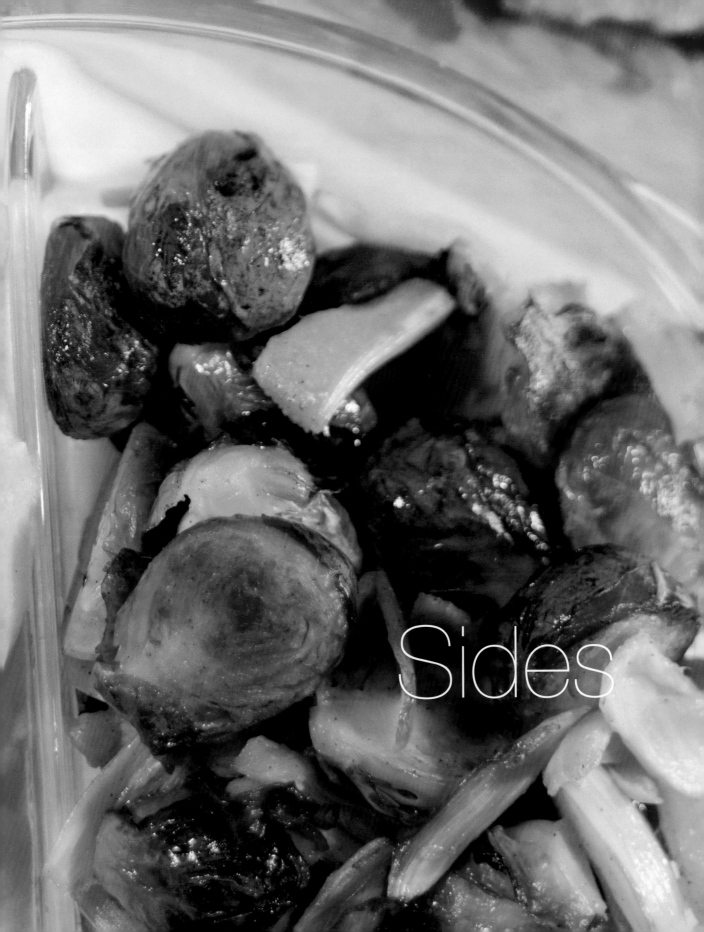

Sides

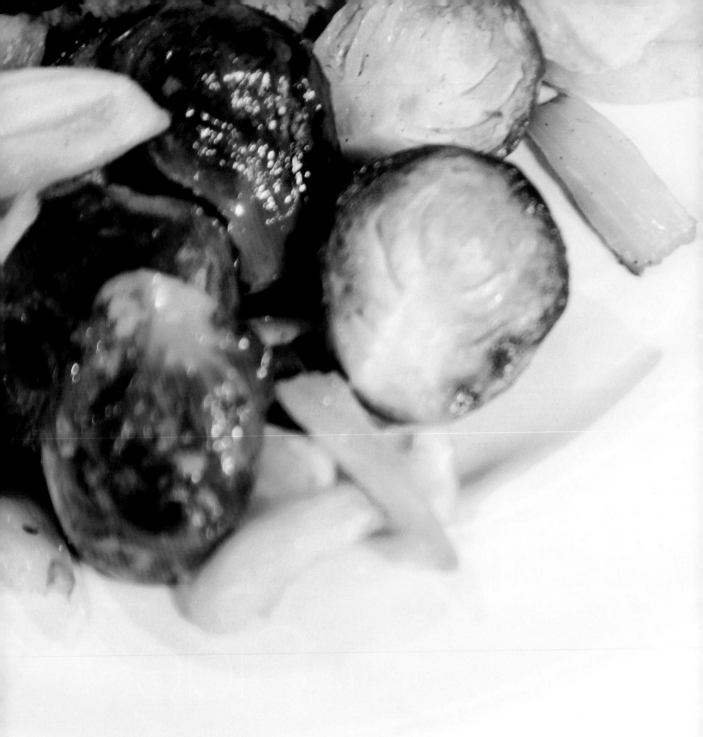

Baked Brussels Sprouts, Fennel, and Garlic

Think beyond canned peas and carrots or frozen tater tots. When you're in the grocery store, step away from the freezer section and into the produce department. Fresh vegetables and herbs can be cooked hundreds of ways to produce myriad flavors. Prepared well, a vegetable side dish is anything but boring.

The recipes in this section can serve to broaden your horizons, *vegetably* speaking. Sides not only compliment the meal, but often times make the meal.

Baked Brussels Sprouts, Fennel, and Garlic

Brussels sprouts are part of the same family as cabbage, which is known to have powerful cancer fighting phytonutrients. Caramelized Brussels sprouts and fennel is a great tasting combination.

¼ cup olive oil
1 pound Brussels sprouts, sliced in half
2 large fennel bulbs, sliced into ½ inch strips

3 large cloves garlic, minced
Salt and pepper
Canola oil spray

Preheat oven to 450 degrees F. In a large bowl, combine oil, Brussels sprouts, fennel, and garlic. Toss well to coat with oil. Pour vegetables onto a large, canola oil-sprayed cookie sheet and place in preheated oven. Roast for about 30 minutes, stirring often, until vegetables are soft and caramelized. Salt and pepper to taste. Serve immediately. **Serves 3-4**

Creamed Spinach

I love creamed spinach, but I don't love the fat that's in the traditional variety. This is a low-fat version.

4 tablespoons olive oil
1 medium onion, diced
3 cloves garlic, minced
8 ounces mushrooms, sliced
10 ounces fresh spinach, chopped

1 tablespoon cornstarch
1 cup nonfat milk
1 tablespoon cooking sherry
2 tablespoon low-fat grated Parmesan cheese
Salt and pepper

In a large skillet, sauté the onion in the 2 tablespoons oil until onions are translucent. Add the garlic and mushrooms and cook until the water is out of the mushrooms. Add spinach, and cook until spinach is wilted. Set aside. In another skillet, heat the remaining 2 tablespoons oil over a high heat and whisk in 1 tablespoon cornstarch to form a paste. Quickly whisk in the milk, whisking constantly until thick. Add sherry and mix well. Add the spinach mixture and combine well. Add the Parmesan cheese. Salt and pepper to taste and serve warm. **Serves 3-4**

Baked Tomatoes

4 large tomatoes, chopped in large chunks
3 large leaves fresh basil, chopped
¼ cup fresh chopped flat-leaf parsley

1 tablespoon olive oil
Olive oil spray
Salt and pepper

Preheat oven to 375 degrees F. Spray a shallow baking dish with olive oil spray. In a large bowl, mix all of the ingredients together, except olive oil spray and salt and pepper. Place in the baking dish. Bake uncovered for about 45 minutes, stirring occasionally until most of the water has baked off and tomatoes are thick. Salt and pepper to taste. **Serves 3-4**

Corn Rice

Get your veggies in any way you can. This dish not only helps do just that, but it also makes plain rice much more interesting.

1 cup brown rice, uncooked
2 cups vegetable broth
1 tablespoon olive oil
1 small onion, chopped

1 (15 ounce) can sweet corn, drained
½ cup fresh chopped flat-leaf parsley
Salt and pepper

Cook rice according to package directions, using 2 cups vegetable broth instead of 2 cups water While rice is cooking, using a small skillet, sauté the onion in the olive oil until onion is translucent, about 10 minutes.

When rice is finished cooking, add the onions, corn, and parsley to the rice while the rice is still warm. Mix well. Salt and pepper to taste.

Serves 3-4

Carrot Mashed Potatoes

This is a good way to take mashed potatoes up to the next level. Carrots have been shown in studies to reduce a number of different cancers including lung, stomach, intestine, bladder, prostate, and breast.

2 pounds peeled potatoes,
cut in 1 inch chunks
2 large peeled carrots, cut in 1 inch chunks

½ cup nonfat sour cream
½ cup nonfat milk
Salt and pepper

Place the potatoes and carrots in a pot and cover with just enough cold water to cover the vegetables. Bring to a boil, reduce heat, and simmer until the vegetables are tender (about 15-20 minutes).

When the vegetables are tender, drain the water from the pot, then place the pot back on the burner for 1 minute to cook off the remaining water and dry the vegetables. Remove from heat.

Add sour cream and milk to potatoes and carrots. Mash until desired consistency. Salt and pepper to taste. Serve while hot.

Serves 3-4

Curried Greens and Rice

Dark greens, curry, garlic, and tomatoes are all cancer fighting foods. Get your green on, and mix them together in this Indian-spiced side dish.

2 cups brown rice, uncooked
4 cups vegetable broth or fat-free chicken broth
2 tablespoons curry powder
2 tablespoons olive oil
1 medium onion, diced
3 cloves garlic, minced

1 tablespoon turmeric
1 (15.5 ounce) can diced tomatoes
1 tablespoon raw brown sugar
1 tablespoon tomato paste
1 pound greens, washed and chopped
Salt and pepper

Cook the brown rice according to package directions using the 4 cups of broth instead of water, and adding 1 tablespoon curry powder to broth as it cooks. Set aside. Heat the olive oil in a large skillet. Add the onion, and sauté over medium heat, stirring often until onion is soft and gets some color. Add the garlic, 1 tablespoon curry powder, turmeric, tomatoes, brown sugar, and tomato paste. Turn heat down, and continue to simmer for 5-10 minutes.

Add the cooked rice to the tomato mixture and stir well. Add the greens, a little bit at a time, mixing in each small bunch. The greens will wilt into the mixture. Continue to cook for another 10 minutes, stirring often. Salt and pepper to taste.

Serves 6

Mushroom Rice

Even the simple button mushrooms have been found to reduce the risk of breast cancer and prostate cancer. Why not use them whenever possible? This easy recipe turns ordinary rice into a dinner treat.

1 cup brown rice, uncooked
2 cups mushroom broth
1 tablespoon olive oil
1 small onion, chopped

½ pound mushrooms (any variety), chopped
½ cup chopped flat-leaf parsley
Salt and pepper

Cook rice according to package directions using mushroom broth instead of water. In a small skillet, sauté the onion in the olive oil. When onion is translucent, add the mushrooms and cook until water is out of the mushrooms, about 10 minutes. Add the onions and mushrooms to the rice while the rice is still warm. Mix well. Add parsley and toss well. Salt and pepper to taste.

Serves 3-4

Roasted Vegetables

This dish is great comfort food, and the smell of the roasting vegetables will permeate the house and put a smile on your family's faces. In addition, every vegetable in this dish has been shown to have cancer fighting properties!

4 beets, peeled and cut in 1 inch pieces
⅓ cup + 2 tablespoons olive oil
1 butternut squash, skin and seeds removed, cut in 1 inch cubes
1 red pepper, seeded and diced
1 sweet potato, peeled, cut in 1 inch cubes
1 potato, unpeeled, cut in 1 inch cubes
1 large red onion, cut in 1 inch pieces

2 large carrots, peeled and cut in 1 inch pieces
4 cloves garlic, minced
2 tablespoons thyme, chopped finely
2 tablespoons rosemary, chopped finely
¼ cup flat-leaf parsley, chopped
Canola oil spray
Salt and pepper

Preheat oven to 450 degrees F.

In a small bowl, mix together the beets and 2 tablespoons olive oil. Place the beets onto a canola oil-sprayed baking sheet and spread out. Place in preheated oven.

Place all of the remaining ingredients (except parsley, salt, and pepper) into a large bowl and mix well until all of the vegetables are well coated with remaining oil and herbs. Spread the vegetables out evenly in a large, canola oil-sprayed roasting pan. Place in preheated oven.

Roast the pan of vegetables and the beets for about 45 minutes to 1 hour until vegetables and beets are tender. Turn often with spoon or spatula to ensure that vegetables and beets brown on all sides.

When all of the vegetables and beets are tender, remove from oven. Add the parsley. Mix the beets and the pan vegetables together gently to avoid all of the vegetables becoming "beet red." Salt and pepper to taste. Serve hot or cold.

Serves 4-6

Mexican-Flavored Potatoes

The potato has gotten a bad name in some nutrition circles, but it shouldn't have. The potato isn't bad for you. It's the way it's cooked (fried) or toppings that are heaped on (sour cream and butter) that are unhealthy, not the potato itself. Potatoes are actually very high in antioxidants, Vitamin C, and iron.

2 pounds unpeeled potatoes, any type
1 medium onion, diced
1 small red pepper, seeded and diced
3 cloves garlic, minced
¼ cup chopped jarred pimento, drained well
¼ cup olive oil

1½ teaspoons cumin
1 teaspoon chili powder
¼ cup chopped fresh cilantro
Canola oil spray
Salt and pepper

Preheat the oven to 400 degrees F. Cut the potatoes into 1 inch chunks. Place the cut potatoes in a bowl, along with the onion, red pepper, garlic, pimento, olive oil, cumin, and chili powder. Toss well until the potatoes are entirely coated with oil and spices.

Spread the potato/pepper mixture onto a large baking sheet sprayed with canola oil spray. Place in the preheated oven for 1 hour, or until done. Turn the potatoes over a couple of times with a large spoon or spatula during the roasting process to ensure that the potatoes brown on all sides. Top with cilantro when the potatoes come out of the oven. Salt and pepper to taste. Serve hot.

Serves 4-6

Indian Spiced Brown Rice

Just a little spice and a few raisins can really pick up ordinary rice. Turmeric has been used as a spice for hundreds of years, and its medicinal properties are many. Turmeric is known for its anti-inflammatory properties and in labs has proven to help fight several types of cancer.

4 cups vegetable stock
2 cups brown rice, uncooked
2 cloves garlic, minced
1 teaspoon curry

1 teaspoon turmeric
1 cup raisins
Salt and pepper

In a medium pot, combine vegetable stock and rice. Add garlic, curry, turmeric, and raisins. Mix well. Bring to a boil, then cover, reduce heat, and simmer about 40 minutes. Salt and pepper to taste.

Serves 3-4

Green Rice

Serving green rice is another way to get some extra veggies in and make the dinner or picnic just a little more interesting. This is a versatile dish as you can use any greens you like, and you can also vary your spices. Got some fresh herbs? Oregano, tarragon, basil? Toss 'em in.

2 tablespoons olive oil
3 green onions, chopped
2 cloves garlic, minced
2 cups fresh spinach, chopped
4½ cups vegetable stock

2 cups brown rice, uncooked
½ cup chopped chives
½ cup chopped fresh flat-leaf parsley
Salt and pepper

In a large skillet, sauté the onions in the olive oil over a medium-high heat, until onions are translucent. Add garlic and spinach and sauté until spinach is wilted. Place spinach in a blender with 2 cups vegetable stock and blend until smooth. In a medium pot, combine spinach with remaining vegetable stock and rice. Mix well. Bring to a boil, cover, reduce heat, and simmer until rice is of desired texture (about 20 minutes). When rice is finished, add herbs. Salt and pepper to taste.

Serves 3-4

Horseradish Twice-Baked Potatoes

This is a really tasty side dish but does take a little more effort than a plain baked potato. The recipe calls for *Onion Butter*, but if you haven't made a batch, you can omit it and the potato will still taste great. If you omit the *Onion Butter*, just add a little more milk to get a thinner consistency.

2 large baking potatoes
¼ cup *Onion Butter*
¼ cup nonfat sour cream
2-4 tablespoons nonfat milk
2 teaspoons prepared horseradish

½ teaspoon celery salt
¼ teaspoon cracked black pepper
Paprika
¼ cup *Caramelized Onions with Balsamic Vinegar*

Preheat oven to 350 degrees F. With a fork, prick holes in the potatoes in several places and cook in microwave until done. Potatoes should depress a little when pressed in the center. Carefully, cut the potatoes in half lengthwise and scoop out most of the insides of the potatoes, leaving about 1/8 inch of potato on the skin. Place the potato skins on a small baking sheet. In a bowl, mix the potato inside with *Onion Butter*, sour cream, 2 tablespoons milk, horseradish, and salt and pepper. With a hand mixer, mix until smooth. Add the additional 2 tablespoons of milk if necessary to get desired consistency. Divide the mixture evenly into the 4 potato shells. Sprinkle with paprika. Place into preheated oven for 10-15 minutes until potatoes are hot. Remove from oven and top each potato half with 1 tablespoon *Caramelized Onions*. Serve immediately.

Serves 4

Non Creamed Zucchini and Spinach

Popeye had the right idea downing those cans of spinach. Spinach is a member of the cruciferous family. Studies have shown that eating spinach may decrease your risk of several cancers.

3 tablespoons olive oil
1 large onion, diced
2 cloves garlic, minced
½ cup vegetable broth
2 medium zucchini, chopped

4 cups fresh spinach leaves, chopped
1 tablespoon cornstarch
¼ cup nonfat milk
Juice of one lemon
Salt and pepper

In a large skillet, heat the oil over a medium-high heat. Add the onions and the garlic and cook until the onions are translucent. Add the vegetable broth. Add the zucchini and lower the heat. Cover and simmer until the zucchini are soft. Add the spinach and cook until the spinach is wilted and the vegetable broth is almost gone, leaving the mixture a little moist.

Dissolve cornstarch in milk. Add the cornstarch mixture to the spinach/zucchini mixture and stir well. Spinach/zucchini mixture will begin the thicken. Add the juice of the lemon. Salt and pepper to taste. Mix well and serve immediately.

Serves 3-4

Pumpkin Puree

I like to make this as a side dish when pumpkin is in season. Carving pumpkins are not as tasty as the smaller pumpkins or the white pumpkins. This recipe is a simple yet elegant autumn treat.

1 white pumpkin
1 cup unsweetened applesauce
¼ teaspoon nutmeg

¼ teaspoon cloves
½ teaspoon cinnamon
Salt and pepper

Preheat oven to 350 degrees F. Cut the top off the pumpkin and scrape out the seeds. Cut the pumpkin in large wedges and place the wedges flesh side down in 9" x 13" baking dish that has a small amount of water in the bottom. Cover with aluminum foil and place in the preheated oven. Bake for about 1 hour until the flesh of the pumpkin is soft. (You can test it by poking the flesh with a sharp knife.) Remove from the oven and allow to cool. When pumpkin is cool enough to touch, scoop out the pumpkin flesh and place into a food processor with all other ingredients. Blend until smooth. Salt and pepper to taste. Serve hot.

Serves 3-4

Pumpkin Mashed Potatoes

Pumpkins aren't just for Halloween Jack-O-Lanterns and Thanksgiving pies. They're also a super nutritious vegetable full of beta-carotene, a powerful antioxidant. Mixing some into some mashed potatoes makes the mashed potatoes less boring and may help reduce the risk of some cancers.

1 small pumpkin
2 pounds peeled potatoes, quartered
2 large peeled sweet potatoes, cut in large chunks
½ cup nonfat or soy milk

¼ cup nonfat sour cream
Pinch of nutmeg
Pinch of ginger
¼ cup chopped fresh flat-leaf parsley
Salt and pepper

Preheat oven to 350 degrees F. Cut the top off the pumpkin and scrape out the seeds. Cut the pumpkin in large wedges and place wedges, flesh side down, in a 9" x 13" baking dish that has a small amount of water in the bottom. Cover with aluminum foil and place in the preheated oven. Bake for about 1 hour, or until the flesh of the pumpkin is soft. Allow to cool. Scoop out pumpkin flesh and set aside.

While pumpkin is baking, boil white potatoes and sweet potatoes until soft, then drain. Place all ingredients (except parsley and salt and pepper) in a food processor and blend until smooth. You might need more or less milk, depending on the size of your potatoes, to get the desired consistency. Stir in parsley by hand. Salt and pepper to taste. Serve immediately.

Serves 4-6

Sautéed Broccoli with Garlic

This recipe is incredibly simple and takes ordinary broccoli to a gourmet level. This is one of my favorite ways to do broccoli, or any vegetable, for that matter.

1 large bunch broccoli, cut in small florets.
3 tablespoons olive oil

3 large cloves garlic, minced
Salt and pepper

Steam the broccoli to al dente texture. Do not overcook. They will get cooked further when sautéed.

Dry the broccoli well. Heat the oil in a large skillet. Add the broccoli and sauté on a medium-high heat, stirring constantly for 2 minutes. Add the garlic and continue to sauté until the broccoli softens and browns, about 5-6 minutes. Remove from heat. Salt and pepper to taste and serve hot.

Serves 3-4

Smashed Kale and Onion Potatoes

Kale is a very healthy vegetable that gets ignored by many. I happen to like the taste of it and include it in my salads, but stashing it into your mashed potatoes is a great way to get your kale in. Kale is from the same family as cabbage, and studies have shown that people who eat a lot of cruciferous vegetables have a lower incident of several different types of cancer.

2 pounds unpeeled potatoes, quartered
3 tablespoons olive oil
1 onion, chopped finely
3 large cloves garlic, minced
1 bunch kale, stems removed, chopped

¼ cup nonfat sour cream
½ cup nonfat or soy milk
¼ cup chopped flat-leaf parsley
Salt and pepper

Fill a large pot with water and place potatoes in the pot. Bring water to a boil and reduce heat. Simmer until potatoes are tender. In a large skillet, heat olive oil and add onions. Cook slowly until onions are translucent. Add garlic and chopped kale and cook until kale is wilted. Set aside. Drain water from the potatoes and mash well. Add milk and sour cream and mash until desired consistency. You might need more or less milk depending on the size of the potatoes. Add parsley and kale/onion mixture. Stir to blend. Salt and pepper to taste. Serve hot.

Serves 3-4

Squash Casserole

2 tablespoons olive oil
1 large onion, diced
1 clove garlic, crushed
3 large zucchini, diced
4 large yellow squash, diced
½ cup *Yogurt Cheese* (drained in the refrigerator for 24 hours)

½ cup shredded cheese (part-skim mozzarella, veggie, or soy)
½ cup Panko bread crumbs
Canola oil spray
Salt and pepper

Preheat oven to 350 degrees F. In a large skillet, heat olive oil over medium heat. Add onion and sauté until onion is transparent. Add garlic, diced zucchini, and squash and cook until water is out of the squash, about 30 minutes. Add *Yogurt Cheese* and shredded cheese. Continue cooking until absolutely all of the water from the vegetables and the *Yogurt Cheese* is out of the mixture (or the casserole, once baked, will separate and be watery). Salt and pepper to taste. Pour into a canola oil-sprayed 2-quart baking dish and top with Panko bread crumbs. Bake for 20 minutes.

Serves 3-4

Sautéed Green Beans

This recipe is so easy to prepare, and it adds an extra layer of flavor to green beans, rendering them something special instead of just ho hum steamed beans.

1 pound fresh green beans
2 cloves garlic, minced

2 tablespoons extra-virgin olive oil
Salt and pepper

Snap the ends off of the green beans. Steam the green beans to an al dente texture. Do not overcook as they will get further cooking when sautéed. Dry the green beans well. Heat the oil in a large skillet. Add the green beans and sauté on a medium-high heat, stirring constantly for 2 minutes. Add the garlic and continue to sauté until the beans soften and begin to brown (about 5-6 minutes). Remove from heat. Salt and pepper to taste and serve hot. **Serves 3-4**

Sautéed Greens and Tomatoes

These greens taste almost creamed when cooked down with tomatoes.

1 large onion, diced
2 tablespoons olive oil
1 pound mushrooms, diced
2 large garlic cloves, crushed

8 cups greens, chopped
2 large tomatoes, diced
Salt and pepper

In a large skillet, sauté onion in olive oil until slightly translucent. Add mushrooms and sauté until water is out of the mushrooms, about 5 minutes. When onions and mushrooms are cooked, add crushed garlic and greens. Sauté until greens are wilted, about 3 minutes. Add tomatoes and lower heat to very low. Cook greens down, stirring occasionally, until almost all of the water has cooked out (leave some water; you want the greens moist). Salt and pepper to taste. **Serves 3-4**

Sautéed Mushrooms and Kale

Kale has been gaining in popularity and rightfully so. It could be one of the healthiest vegetables that exist.

3 tablespoons olive oil
1 pound mushrooms, sliced
1 clove garlic, crushed

1 large bunch kale, chopped
Salt and pepper

In a large skillet, heat olive oil over medium heat and add sliced mushrooms. Cook until water is out of the mushrooms, about 10 minutes. Stir in garlic. Add kale. Stir until kale wilts. Salt and pepper to taste. **Serves 3-4**

Sweet and Sour Red Cabbage

All cruciferous vegetables are great for fighting cancer, but red cabbage in particular has been shown in studies to help fight several different kinds of cancer, including breast, lung, stomach, and colon. This is a very tasty side dish to almost any meal. It's a treat, whether eaten hot or cold.

1 tablespoon canola oil
1 red onion, diced
1 small head red cabbage, cored and diced into 1 inch pieces
3 large apples, cored and diced
1½-2½ cups water
¾ cup apple cider vinegar

¼ cup raw brown sugar
¼ cup raisins
2 tablespoons pickling spice, tied up in cheesecloth or a coffee filter
2 tablespoons cornstarch
2 tablespoons water
Salt and pepper

In a large skillet, brown the onion in the canola oil. Place the rest of the ingredients in the skillet (except salt and pepper) and bring to a boil. Liquid should just cover all of the ingredients in the skillet, so adjust the water accordingly. Lower the heat to a simmer and cover. Cook for about 1 hour, until all ingredients are soft. Remove the spice bag and blend the cabbage quickly with an electric hand blender. Be careful not to puree the mixture but allow chunks to remain. Dissolve cornstarch in water. Turn heat under cabbage/apple mixture to high. Mix in cornstarch mixture, stirring constantly to thicken and avoid burning. Cabbage should thicken almost immediately. Remove from heat. Salt and pepper to taste. Serve hot.

Serves 6-8

Mexican-Flavored Beans

This recipe came out of the kitchen of a little Mexican restaurant I frequent. One of the cooks was nice enough to share it with me, and I'm passing it on.

16 ounces dry pinto beans, rinsed well
1 large onion, cut in 1 inch chunks
8 cups vegetable broth
3 large cloves garlic, crushed

1 teaspoon salt
1 teaspoon cumin
½ teaspoon pepper
1 teaspoon jalapeno, chopped (optional)

Place beans in a medium stock pot and cover with water plus one inch. Bring to a rolling boil. Remove from heat, cover with lid, and allow to rest for one hour. Drain water and place back on stove. Place all other ingredients in the pot and bring to a boil again. Reduce heat as low as possible and partially cover, but allow a little steam to escape. Cook for 4-5 hours until beans are soft and onions dissolved. Add water or broth if necessary. When done, the liquid should still barely cover the beans.

Serves 6

Sweet Potato Air Fries

Sweet potatoes are high in beta-carotene, Vitamin E, fiber, and are fat-free. Who knew something that tastes so good could be so good for us? Although they are not as crispy as ordinary fries, they are just as much of a treat. My family even prefers them!

6 sweet potatoes
3 tablespoon olive oil

Salt and pepper to taste
Canola oil spray

Preheat oven to 400 degrees F. Peel the potatoes and slice them into ¼ inch strips. (Try to cut them uniformly so they bake evenly.) Place the strips in a bowl. Toss them with the olive oil and salt and pepper to coat well. Spray a baking sheet with canola oil spray. Spread the fries out on the baking sheet, so they are evenly spread out on a single layer. (You may need a second baking sheet, depending on the size of the potatoes. Just make sure the potatoes are spread out in a single layer.) Place the sheet or sheets into the oven. Bake for 45-60 minutes. Turn with a spatula once or twice to make sure they brown on all sides. Fries should be crisp on the outside.

Note: If you are short on time, you can par-cook the fries in the microwave first so that they are about ½ cooked, not totally cooked. Then coat with oil and place in the oven. This saves some cooking time.

Serves 3-4

Sweet Potato Hash Browns

The little root vegetable is actually a distant relative to the white potato and is itself a super power food. The sweet potato has been shown to help with everything from constipation to strokes to diabetes. In addition, it's high in beta-carotene, which helps the body fight against free radicals.

3 tablespoons canola oil
1 onion, diced
3 medium peeled sweet potatoes, grated

Salt and pepper
Canola oil spray

In a large skillet or on a griddle, heat the oil and add the onion. Sauté over a medium-high heat until the onion is soft and has some color. Add the sweet potatoes, flattening them out with a spatula. Cook for about 20 minutes, until potatoes are cooked through and the outside is crispy. Flip several times through cooking to ensure the potatoes are browned on both sides. Salt and pepper to taste.

Serves 4

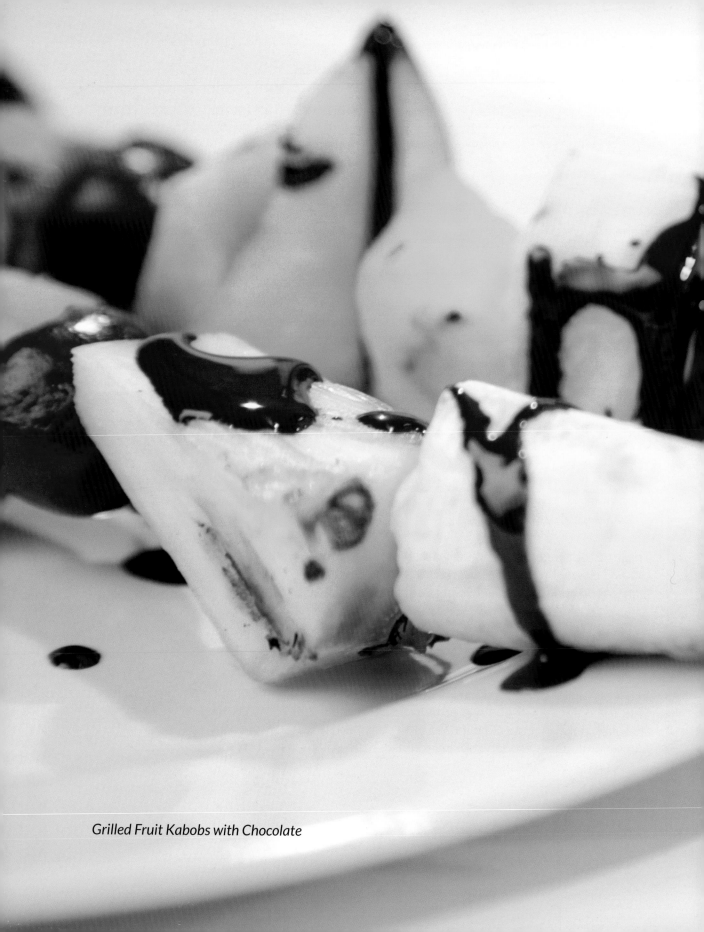

Grilled Fruit Kabobs with Chocolate

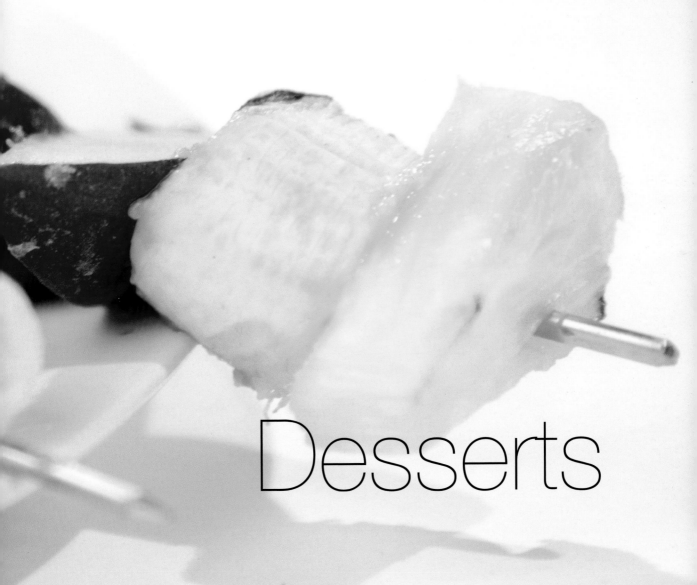

Desserts

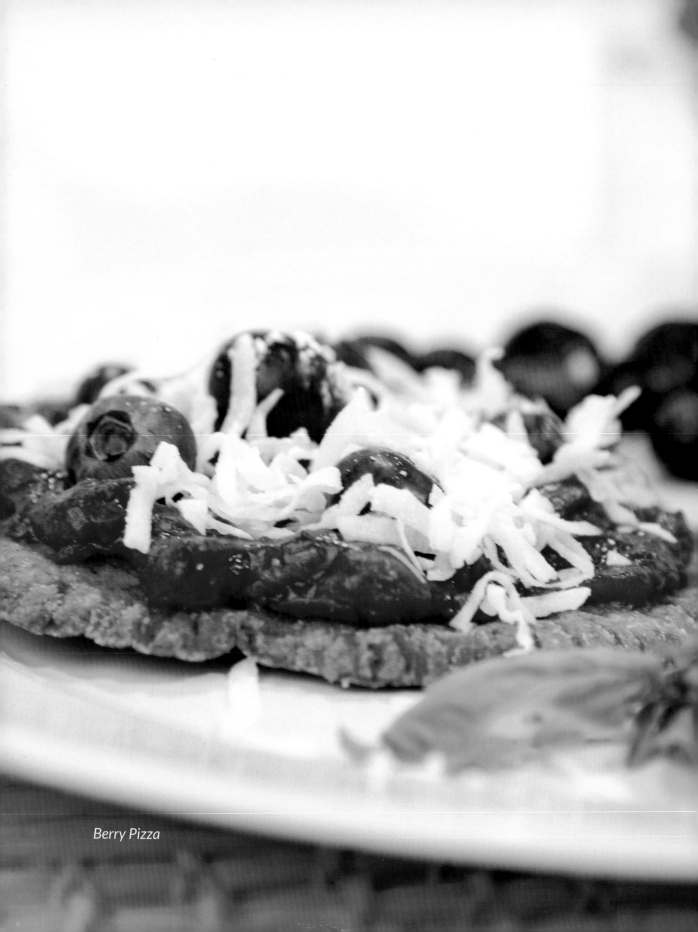

Berry Pizza

Who doesn't like a good dessert? Sadly, most desserts are not among the healthiest things we can eat. Most of the time, they're loaded with unhealthy fats and sugar, and we need to avoid them if we want to stay healthy.

Many of us have at least a bit of a sweet tooth, and a meal just doesn't seem complete without a sweet ending of some sort. The good news is that with a little planning and preparation, and a retraining of our palates (which we can do), we don't have to totally forego feeding that sweet tooth.

Most nights I enjoy just a piece of fruit or a chunk of dark chocolate for dessert, but sometimes, especially if company is coming, I want a little something more.

In this section, I've included a few favorite dessert recipes that are made with fresh fruit, dark chocolate, and nonfat yogurt. They should satisfy your craving for something sweet without causing you too much guilt. You'll be surprised how much your family and guests will appreciate them, too!

Baked Pears

What smells better than baked pears cooking in the oven on an autumn day? This will fill your house with a great aroma and your body with fiber and Vitamin C.

5 firm pears	2 tablespoons chopped walnuts
3 tablespoons maple syrup	2 tablespoons chopped almonds
1 teaspoon cinnamon	Canola oil spray

Preheat oven to 350 degrees F. Spray a cookie sheet with canola oil.

Remove core and cut pears lengthwise into 8 wedges each. In a large bowl, mix pears, syrup, cinnamon, and nuts until well coated. Place pears on sprayed cookie sheet and cook until soft, about 30 minutes.

Serve warm or cold.

Serves 4-6

Berry Pizza

This is a slight variation on a berry pie and, quite frankly, who can resist a fresh berry pie? This is a healthier version than most made to resemble a pizza. Most pie crusts are made with some kind of fat or lard, and that's a diet no-no. This is a cross between a crust and a cookie and is fun to eat as a pizza. Berries are wondrous little fruits that contain phytochemicals and flavonoids.

½ cup whole wheat flour	Zest of one lemon
½ cup low-fat graham crackers, crushed	Juice of one lemon
½ teaspoon salt	¼ cup raw brown sugar (if necessary—taste the berries for sweetness first)
1 teaspoon cinnamon	
¼ cup canola oil	3 tablespoons cornstarch
1 teaspoon raw brown sugar	¼ cup water
3 tablespoons cold water	1 cup of fresh or frozen blueberries
Canola oil spray	2 tablespoons shredded coconut
4 cups fresh strawberries, sliced	

Berry Pizza (cont.)

Preheat oven to 375 degrees F. In a mixing bowl, stir together flour, crushed graham crackers, salt, and cinnamon. Pour in oil and mix with a fork until well blended. Sprinkle cold water on top and mix slightly with fork until dough forms.

Roll dough into a ball and cut into 6 equal pieces. Roll the pieces into balls. One at a time flatten the balls and place each onto a well-floured flat surface for rolling out. Dust the dough on both sides with flour. With a rolling pin, roll each ball out into a 5-inch circle. Flour both sides as you continue to roll to prevent sticking. Don't worry about getting a perfect circle, you can fix that later. Remove each circle with a spatula and place side by side onto a canola oil-sprayed cookie sheet.

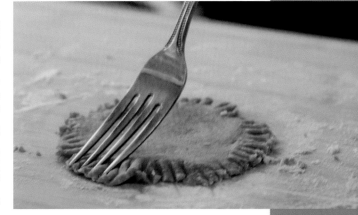

With a fork, working with the tines pointing towards the outside of the circle, go around the edge, pressing toward the center to create a ½ inch crimped edge (*as shown*). While doing this you can reform the circle so that is more round. This procedure of pressing from the outside to the inside is the opposite of what is normally called for, but this is a very crumbly dough and will hold up better this way. Prick the bottom of each circle with a fork several times. Place in a preheated oven for 10-15 minutes. Bake until just firm. This is a darker colored dough. You aren't looking for it to brown, just firm up. Remove from oven and allow to cool.

Place strawberries in a saucepan over medium heat. Add the lemon juice and zest and stir. Cook until the strawberries are soft. Mash slightly to break up the strawberries. Taste the mixture for desired sweetness. Add the raw brown sugar, if needed.

In a small bowl, mix the cornstarch and the water together until dissolved. Increase the heat to high. When the berries begin to boil, add the cornstarch mixture while stirring constantly. Mixture should thicken immediately.

Remove from heat and allow to cool for 10 minutes. Spoon a portion of the strawberries onto each circle, not quite going all the way to the edge, just like sauce on a pizza. Place the blueberries on top of each piece to resemble a healthy sausage topping. Sprinkle one teaspoon of shredded coconut over each piece to resemble cheese. Each piece should look like a miniature pizza. Place in the refrigerator until chilled.

Serves 6

Carrot Cake

With a name like carrot cake, you'd think it would be healthy, wouldn't you? Truth is, most carrot cakes are some of the most fat-laden desserts you can have! This is a healthier, less caloric version of a family favorite.

2 cups white whole wheat flour
1 tablespoon baking soda
1 teaspoon baking powder
2 teaspoons cinnamon
1 teaspoon nutmeg
1 teaspoon salt
3 cups grated carrots

2 egg whites
1 cup *Yogurt Cheese*
1½ cups applesauce
½ cup maple syrup
½ cup chopped walnuts
Canola oil spray

Preheat the oven to 350 degrees F. In a large bowl, mix flour, baking soda, baking powder, cinnamon, nutmeg, and salt. Add the rest of the ingredients (except canola oil spray) and stir until well combined. Pour mixture into a canola oil-sprayed 9"× 13" baking dish. Bake for 40 minutes or until done. Cool thoroughly and then frost with *Faux Yogurt Cream Cheese Topping* (see below).

Serves 6-8

Faux Yogurt Cream Cheese Topping

2 cups *Yogurt Cheese* (drained for 24 hours)
Zest of one orange
1 teaspoon vanilla
2 tablespoons honey

In a medium bowl, gently mix together *Yogurt Cheese*, orange zest, vanilla, and honey. Cover with plastic wrap and place bowl in the refrigerator. Allow to chill and ingredients to meld together for another 1-2 hours.

Chocolate Covered Almonds

8 ounces raw almonds
8 ounces dark chocolate (at least 70% cacao)

Preheat oven to 350 degrees F. Spread out almonds on a baking sheet and place in the preheated oven for 10-15 minutes or until the nuts are nicely toasted. Remove from oven.

Melt chocolate in a double boiler. Remove from heat and add the almonds to the melted chocolate. Stir well, until completely coated.

Using a fork, remove the almonds from the double boiler and place on the wax paper-lined baking sheet. Refrigerate the cookie sheet of almonds until the chocolate hardens. This chocolate has not been tempered, so refrigerate until ready to serve. The chocolate will melt somewhat quickly at room temperature. Don't worry, they go quickly!

Serves 3-4

Chocolate Covered Berries

A diet rich in all kinds of berries may help to reduce your risk of several types of cancers. Dark chocolate (though not milk chocolate or white chocolate) has been shown to be a potent antioxidant. Moderation is key. Dark chocolate still has plenty of calories and fat, so consume in moderation.

    2 cups fresh blueberries, strawberries, blackberries or raspberries, or a combination of all
    1 cup dark chocolate (at least 70% cacao), cut in small pieces

In a double boiler, heat the chocolate and stir until smooth.

If you are using strawberries or blackberries, grab the berries by the top greens and dip into the melted chocolate, or use a fork poked into the top of the berry and dip into the melted chocolate. Place the dipped fruit on top of a sheet of wax paper placed on a cookie sheet.

If you are using blueberries or raspberries, you can dip the blueberries or raspberries one at a time using a toothpick, or drop in several at once. Remove and drop in clusters on the wax paper to set.

When you are finished dipping the berries, place the sheet in the refrigerator to set. The chocolate has not been tempered, so refrigerate until ready to serve—the chocolate will melt quickly at room temperature. These are best if eaten the same day as dipped.

Note: Sliced bananas are great for dipping also!

Serves 3-4

Pear Apple Compote

Pears are high in fiber and high in Vitamin C. This dish is incredibly simple and always gets raves.

    2 cups apple juice, unsweetened   ¼ cup raisins
    3 firm pears, chopped   1 teaspoon cinnamon
    3 apples, chopped   ¼ teaspoon nutmeg
    1 teaspoon vanilla   2 tablespoons chopped walnuts

Place all ingredients in a saucepan and bring to a boil. Lower heat and simmer until most of the liquid evaporates. Mash slightly with a potato masher or a hand held mixer. Serve warm or cold.

Serves 4-6

Fruit Bake

This is a very versatile dessert. I've used winter fruits, but you can really substitute most other fruits—peaches, nectarines, cherries, etc. Eating a diet high in fruits is essential in the battle against cancer. In studies, persons with low fruit and vegetable intake experience about twice the risk of cancer compared to those who have a high intake of fruits and veggies.

2 large apples, cored and diced in 1 inch chunks
2 large pears, cored and diced in 1 inch chunks
½ cup dried apricots, diced
½ cup raisins
Zest of one lemon
Juice of one lemon
2 tablespoons white whole wheat flour
¼ cup chopped walnuts
1 teaspoon cinnamon
½ teaspoon nutmeg
Canola oil spray

Preheat oven to 350 degrees F. In a large bowl, combine all of the fruit with the zest and the juice of the lemon. Add the 2 tablespoons of whole wheat flour, walnuts, cinnamon, and nutmeg and mix well, until fruit is well coated. Pour fruit into a canola oil-sprayed 9" x 13" baking dish. Top with *Oatmeal Topping* and bake for 45 minutes in preheated oven. The top of the fruit should be a little brown. Serve warm.

Serves 6-8

Melted Chocolate

1 cup dark chocolate (at least 70% cacao), cut in small pieces

In a double boiler, place water in the lower pot and heat to simmer.

Place the candy in the top pot of the double boiler and stir until the candy melts and becomes smooth. Be careful not to splash any water into the chocolate in the top of the double boiler or the chocolate will seize and become unusable.

Oatmeal Topping

½ cup rolled oats
¼ cup sliced almonds
2 tablespoons white whole wheat flour
2 tablespoons honey
2 tablespoon light olive oil or canola oil
1 tablespoon vanilla

In a small mixing bowl, combine all ingredients and mix well.

Grilled Fruit Kabobs With Chocolate

This is a fun summer dessert and a great way to use the grill!

2 mangos, peeled and cut in 1 inch pieces
2 bananas, peeled and cut in 1 inch chunks
2 peaches, cut in wedges
1 cup cherries, pitted
½ fresh pineapple, cut in 1 inch chunks

Skewer fruit pieces randomly onto six 12 inch skewers. Place on a clean, medium-high, oiled grill and cook until fruit is soft and caramelized, about 5 minutes on each side. Using a pot holder or oven glove, remove skewers and place on a large platter. Drizzle with the *Melted Chocolate*.

Serves 4

Poached Pears

Pears are a great source of Vitamin C, critical for keeping your immune system functioning well. In addition, studies have shown that one serving of apples or pears a day is associated with a reduced risk of lung cancer in women. Put a pot of poached pears on the stove during the holiday season, or any season for that matter, and enjoy the smell and the smiles throughout the house!

6 firm pears (preferably Bartlett, not Bosc), cored and quartered
4 cups unsweetened apple juice
Juice of 1 lemon

1 teaspoon cinnamon
½ teaspoon ground cloves
1 orange, juice and zest
2 tablespoons chopped walnuts

Place pears in a medium-sized pot. Add the apple juice, orange juice, lemon juice, cinnamon, cloves, and orange zest. Add the walnuts. Simmer on a low heat until the pears are tender (about one hour). For the last 5 minutes of cooking, turn the heat to high to boil down the remaining juice until it reduces to about 1 cup of liquid. Pour a little juice over each pear. Serve warm or cold .

Serves 6

Pumpkin Cheesecake

This cake is an indulgence, but sometimes—especially around the holidays—I have to indulge. This is a semi-healthy indulgence. It is low-fat and contains healthy pumpkin. Pumpkin is an excellent source of beta-carotene, which has been shown to help reduce the risk of many types of cancer.

9 low-fat graham crackers
24 ounces *Yogurt Cheese*
4 egg whites
¼ cup honey
2 cups canned pumpkin, plain
¼ cup raw brown sugar

1 tablespoon pumpkin pie spice
¼ teaspoon ground cloves
¼ teaspoon nutmeg
1 tablespoon vanilla
Canola oil spray

Preheat oven to 325 degrees F. Spray an 8" springform pan with canola oil spray. Place the graham crackers, 1 tablespoon *Yogurt Cheese*, 1 egg white and 1 tablespoon honey into the food processor and pulse until well blended. Spread crumbs on the bottom and 1 inch up the sides of the springform pan. Place into oven and bake for 5 minutes. Place all of the other ingredients in a large bowl and mix until well blended but do not over mix. Spread mixture on top of crumbs in springform pan and bake in preheated oven for about 1½ hours or until cake tests done. Serve with a dollop of *Faux Yogurt Cream Cheese Topping*.

Serves 8

Appendix I

Anti-Cancer Foods and the Studies that Support Their Benefits

The food studies below have been graded using the following criteria:

    A   High-quality randomized controlled trial (RCT) or High-quality meta-analysis (quantitative systematic review)

    B   Nonrandomized clinical trial; Nonquantitative systematic review; Lower quality RCT; Clinical cohort study; Case-control study; Historical control; or Epidemiologic study

    C   Consensus or expert opinion,

    D   Anecdotal evidence; In vitro or animal research

At the close of the Appendix I, you will find a glossary of the terms used that will clearly explain the grading criteria.

You will note that many of the studies below are rated with a **(D)**. That doesn't mean that the study almost "failed." Rather, it means that it was based on anecdotal evidence, or conducted in a laboratory on human cells or perhaps using mice or rats as subjects, but not human beings. Studies conducted on human beings are clinical trials, and are extremely expensive and complicated and take years to complete. There are four phases to a clinical trial; all are overseen by the FDA and are extremely time consuming and complex. Because of their expense, the cost of producing a clinical trial is out of reach for all but the deepest pockets. Funding for clinical research can come from federal government entities such as the National Institute of Health and the Department of Veterans Affairs, or from foundations and medical institutions, but, most of the time, flows from those entities that will be best able to reap the monetary gains from their results–pharmaceutical companies looking to discover and test drugs and supplement manufacturers wishing to sell their products. Studies on cancer-fighting foods are simply not part of their business objectives.

In addition, studies performed in other countries often do not conform to the stringent protocols or criteria required in the United States and hence may not be graded as high.

Much of the food research is done at Universities and funded in part by cancer organizations such as the National Cancer Institute (NCI) or the American Institute for Cancer Research (AICR) who are seeking to get answers to cancer prevention. The grading of A, B, C, or D does not mean "pass" or "fail" then, but rather the extent to which the study was taken. Obviously it is easier, less expensive, and quicker to produce a study with mice than with humans. When the opportunity arises to make the same billions from artichokes, for example, as from drugs, then these studies will be undertaken. In the meantime, the myriad D studies are what we have to work with. Remember that even though a study may have been graded D, it could have been extremely successful, showing very promising results within the laboratory. Grade D notwithstanding, there is still an overwhelming amount of evidence that suggests foods can help prevent cancer.

Apples — The *British Journal of Nutrition* reported in September of 2008 that increasing the compound quercetin, found in onions and apples, may reduce the chance of developing **colon** cancer by 50 per cent. **(D)**

In 2008, researchers at Cornell University's Institute for Comparative and Environmental Toxicology published six studies that showed apples slow down the growth of aggressive **breast** cancer tumors. **(D)**

Artichokes — In a study reported in 2000 at Germany's University of Georgia-Augusta, scientists found that phytochemicals in artichokes blocked chemicals (PSA) in the body that led to **prostate** cancer. **(D)**

A 2008 study reported in *Nutrition and Cancer* showed that properties of polyphenolic extracts from artichokes attacked human **hepatoma (liver** cancer) cells. **(D)**

A 2007 study from researchers at the United States Department of Agriculture found that artichokes ranked seventh in total antioxidant capacity per serving out of more than 1000 common foods. **(C)**

Asparagus — In 2002, studies conducted by the Institute for Cancer Prevention made a preliminary determination that asparagus, the food containing the highest concentrations of the antioxidant glutathione may be very effective in strengthening immune systems against the development of cancer. **(D)**

In 2010, *The Journal of the American Medical Association* reported on a study done in France, involving 385,747 research subjects from 10 European countries. The scientists concluded, "Our results suggest that above-median serum measures of both B6 and methionine, assessed on average five years prior to disease onset, are associated with a reduction of at least 50% on the risk of developing **lung** cancer. An additional association for serum levels of folate was present, that when combined with B6 and methionine, was associated with a two-thirds lower risk of **lung** cancer." Asparagus contains both Vitamin B6 and folate. Foods that contain methionine include poultry, fish, cottage cheese, peanuts, beans, eggs, garlic, lentils, onions, yogurt and sesame seeds. **(B)**

Barley — In a study published in 2007 in the *International Journal of Epidemiology*, conductors of the UK Women's Cohort Study found that participants who ate a diet richest in whole grains such as barley cut their risk of developing **breast** cancer by more than half. **(B)**

In a Western New York Exposures and **Breast** Cancer (WEB) study involving 1,122 women, aged 35–79 years, diagnosed with **breast** cancer between 1996 and 2001, diet in the 12–24 months before diagnosis was assessed with an extensive food frequency questionnaire, and lignan intake was calculated. Postmenopausal women who consumed the most lignans had a significantly lower risk of dying from **breast** cancer than women who ate only small amounts of lignan-containing foods (barley being one of them). **(B)**

A 2007 issue of the *Journal of Agricultural and Food Chemistry* reported on a Swedish study comparing men with **prostate** cancer against a control of healthy men without cancer. Researchers determined that the consumption of lignans, phytonutrients found in barley, raised blood levels of enterolactone. Men with the highest levels of enterolactone were 82% less likely to have **prostate** cancer. **(B)**

Beets — In a Russian study reported in the international scientific journal *Vopr Pitan* in 1993, scientists found that beet juice inhibited the growth of cancer-causing chemicals produced in the stomach from the nitrates found in many processed foods. **(D)**

In a study published in 2002 in the *Journal of Agricultural and Food Chemistry*, University of Wisconsin researchers conducted experiments using mouse liver cells that model the function of human liver cells. They determined that pigments present in red beets boost levels of enzymes that help to detoxify cancer-causing substances and eliminate them from the body, thus supporting cancer prevention. **(D)**

Berries — The American Association for Cancer Research reported in November 2008 that The Cleveland Clinic, in cooperation with Ohio State University and the Central Ohio Compounding Pharmacy, had undertaken a study that showed that blackberries prevent **colon** cancer in rodents. As of this writing, they are engaged in clinical trials that they hope will show the same outcome for humans. **(D)**

Blackberries — Blueberries, Strawberries, Raspberries, Researchers from UCLA's Center for Human Nutrition tested a wide range of berries rich in antioxidants, including blueberries, strawberries, and raspberries, and determined they had the ability to inhibit the growth of human **oral**, **prostate**, **breast**, and **colon** cancer cells. **(D)**

Black Raspberries — *Cancer Prevention Research* reported in 2001 on a study conducted at Ohio State Comprehensive Cancer Center on rats, showing that anthocyanins found in black raspberries may inhibit the growth of cancer cells of the **esophagus** and **throat**. **(D)**

Cancer Prevention Research in November 2010 reported on a study conducted at the University of Illinois at Chicago and found that a black raspberry-supplemented diet produced protective effects in the **intestine**, **colon** and **rectum** and inhibited tumor formation in mice. **(D)**

Blueberries — According to the AICR's report, *Food, Nutrition, Physical Activity, and the Prevention of Cancer: A Global Perspective*, blueberries contain a group of phenolic compounds called anthocyanosides. Scientists believe these may be the most potent antioxidants that have so far been identified. **(C)**

Strawberries and Raspberries — According to the AICR's report, *Food, Nutrition, Physical Activity, and the Prevention of Cancer: A Global Perspective*, strawberries and raspberries in particular are rich in a phytochemical called ellagic acid. The report states that studies have shown its ability to prevent **skin**, **bladder**, **lung**, **esophagus**, and **breast** cancers. It acts as an antioxidant and slows the reproduction of cancer cells. **(C)**

Carrots — A European study reported on in a 2005 issue of the *Journal of Agricultural and Food Chemistry* found that the chemical falcarinol, found in carrots, accounted for a one third reduction in cancer development in rats. **(D)**

Also, see Yellow-orange Vegetables and Fruits and Root Vegetables below.

Chocolate (Dark) — A Harvard University study reported in 2006 that the flavanols in cacao act as anti-cancer agents. A 10-year comparison was made of the deaths of Kuna Indians in Panama to those of the San Blas Islands Indians off Panama's coast. The latter group drank 4 to 5 cups of cacao water a day, while the former drank none. Cacao drinkers had a 630% lower risk of death from cancer. **(C)**

A 2008 research study conducted at Georgetown University Medical Center using a chemical called GECGC, which is based on a compound found in cacao beans, has determined that cacao can slow the growth of and perhaps prevent **colon** cancer. The lab experiment on human **colon** cancer cells slowed their growth by half, and most of the tumor cells were damaged. **(D)**

Citrus — In 2010, the *International Journal of Cancer* reported on a study performed in Japan involving over 42,000 adults that showed that consuming citrus daily was associated with a 17% reduced risk of all cancers, particularly in those subjects who also drank a cup of green tea on a daily basis. **(B)**

A 2005 report from Texas A&M University's Vegetable and Fruit Improvement Center on experiments performed on cancer cells with limonoids, compounds found in citrus fruits, shows that limonoids cause apoptosis, or destruction of cancer cells. Researchers say that these limonoids may prevent cancer from forming, slow the growth of existing cancer, or kill existing cancer cells. **(D)**

Complex Carbohydrates — The American Institute for Cancer Research recommends that we eat about 20 to 30 ounces of complex carbohydrates every day. The WCRF/AICR 2007 second report grades foods containing dietary fiber as Probable for decreasing the risk of **colorectum** cancer and Limited-suggestive for decreasing the risk of **esophagus** cancer. **(C)**

Cruciferous Vegetables — *The Journal of Nutrition* reported in March 2008 on a study done at the Department of Food Science and Nutrition, University of Minnesota. The study indicated that fresh, but not lyophilized (freeze dried), cruciferous vegetables reduced **colon** cancer risk in rats. **(D)**

The Lancelot published a study in 2005 from the International Agency for Cancer Research. The study, done in Lyon, France, found eating cruciferous vegetables at least once a week cut cancer risk for people with inactive versions of two genes, carried by 70% of people. Paul Brennan, lead author of the research letter, stated random trials to absolutely confirm the findings would be expensive and time consuming. He also stated that in the meantime including cabbage, kale, Brussels sprouts, broccoli or turnips in your diet at least once a week may help reduce your risk of developing **lung** cancer. **(B)**

Broccoli and Cauliflower — A study reported in the December 2008 Proceedings of the National Academy of Sciences confirmed the chemical compound Indole-3-Carbinol (I3C), found in broccoli and other cruciferous vegetables, was successful in arresting the development of **breast** cancer. **(D)**

A 2007 U.S. and Canadian study reported in the *Journal of the National Cancer Institute* reported that a high intake of cruciferous vegetables, including broccoli and cauliflower, may be associated with reduced risk of aggressive **prostate** cancer, particularly extraprostatic disease. **(B)**

Cabbage — A study done in Sweden, noted in the *Journal of the American Medical Association*, June 2001, found that women who consumed Brassica vegetables had significant reduction in **breast** cancer risk. The study found that by consuming 1 to 2 servings of Brassica vegetables per day, women could lower their risk of **breast** cancer by as much as 20-40%. **(C)**

A study by the Department of Pharmaceutical Sciences of North Dakota State University, Fargo published in the June 2009 issue of *Cancer Prevention Research*, found that a compound called diindolylmethane, which the stomach produces when it consumes cruciferous vegetables such as cabbage and broccoli, may protect against **colon** cancer. (D)

A study, published in *Cancer Research* in 2006, performed by Rutgers University scientists examined the chemopreventative efficacy of phenethyl isothiocyanate (a cancer chemopreventive constituent of cruciferous vegetables). The results of the study confirmed that phenethyl isothiocyanate inhibits the growth of **prostate** cancer cells in mice. **(D)**

Kale — A 2005 study reported in *Molecular Cancer Therapeutics* found that the sulforaphane, formed when kale is chopped or chewed, triggers an enzyme that helps to clear carcinogens from the body. This function has been shown to inhibit the growth of cancer cells, especially **colon** cancer cells. **(D)**

A study done at Channing Laboratory at Brigham and Women's Hospital and reported in the November 15, 2007 issue of the *International Journal of Cancer* involved analyzed data on 66,384 participants of the Nurses' Health Study. The analyzed data showed the greater the consumption of kaempferol (a type of flavonoid that the nurses got mostly from tea, broccoli, and kale), the lower their chance of developing **ovarian** cancer. **(B)**

Red Cabbage — A study conducted by the Department of Agriculture's Agricultural Research Service (ARS) and published in the *Journal of Agricultural and Food Chemistry* in March of 2005 found that red cabbage contained 36 different varieties of anthocyanins, a class of flavonoids that have been linked to cancer protection. Anthocyanins have been shown to exhibit anticarcinogenic activity against multiple cancer cell types in vitro and tumor types in vivo according to an article published in Cancer Letters in October of 2008. **(D)**

A study conducted by the Fred Hutchinson Cancer Research Center reported in January 2000 that although a diet including significant servings of all vegetables was associated with fighting cancer risk, the strongest reduction of risk of **prostate** cancer was associated with eating cruciferous vegetables like broccoli and red cabbage. **(B)**

Green Tea — A University of Texas M. D. Anderson Cancer Center study reported in November of 2009 established that the polyphenols in extracts from green tea showed promise as a cancer prevention agent for **oral** cancer in patients with a pre-malignant condition known as **oral leukoplakia**. The researchers found over half of the **oral leukoplakia** patients who took the extract had a clinical response. The green tea extract also showed an improvement in a number of biomarkers that may play an important role in predicting cancer growth. While the findings were very encouraging, they were not conclusive and researchers cautioned that further testing is necessary. **(A)**

Proteomics reported in February 2009 that Green Tea Extract alters the levels of many proteins involved in growth, motility, and apoptosis of certain **lung** cancer cells (A549 cells) **(D)**

Herbs and Spices — The June, 2003, *The Journal of Nutrition* reported on Norway's The Norwegian Crop Research Institute, Oslo's Institute for Nutrition Research, Faculty of Medicine, University of Oslo and Japan's Department of Anatomy, Akita University School of Medicine, Pharmaceutical Company, Tokyo's studies that the dried herbs oregano, sage, peppermint, garden thyme, lemon balm, clove, allspice, and cinnamon all contained very high concentrations of antioxidants. Of the dried culinary herbs tested, oregano, sage, peppermint, garden thyme, lemon balm, clove, allspice and cinnamon all contained very high concentrations of antioxidants. The researchers concluded that in a normal diet, intake of herbs may contribute significantly to the total intake of plant antioxidants and might be an even better source of dietary antioxidants than other foods such as fruits, berries, cereals and vegetables. **(D)**

Cilantro/Coriander — In 2009, the journal *Chemico-Biological Interactions* reported on research being performed with Linalool, an essential oil extracted from coriander. Linalool was found to completely eradicate a type of **liver** cancer in really low concentrations. **(D)**

A study from the University of Kerala, India, reported in 2000, showed that feeding coriander seeds to mice with induced **colon** cancer showed a marked effect in the decrease of "bad lipids" and the increase of "good lipids." Thus, coriander acts as a protector against the negative effects of lipid metabolism in **colon** cancer. **(D)**

Cumin — The *Journal of Food Protection* reported in 2001 a study in which cumin proved to protect lab animals from developing **stomach** or **liver** cancer. This may be attributed to the fact that cumin is known to enhance the liver's detoxification enzymes, and is a scavenger for free radicals. **(D)**

A widely noted study by the Cancer Institute in Madras, India showed cumin blocked 83% of chromosome damage created by cancer-causing chemicals. **(D)**

Curcumin — The *Journal of Nutritional Biochemistry* in July 2011 cited a Brazilian study where researchers investigated curcumin's effect on glioblastoma cancer cells. The results found that tumor growth was prevented in cultured human cancer cells, and brain tumors decreased in 81% of the mice. Normal cells were not affected. **(D)**

A study conducted at the University of Texas, published in the September 2005 Biochemical Pharmacology, suggests that even when **breast** cancer is already present, curcumin can help slow the spread of **breast** cancer cells to the lungs in mice. **(D)**

Fennel — Researchers reported in the June 2000 edition of the journal *Oncogene* that fennel contains the chemical compound anetole. Their results demonstrated that anethole inhibits TNF-induced cellular responses, which may explain its role in suppression of inflammation and carcinogenesis. **(D)**

The Biological and Pharmaceutical Bulletin in January of 2011 published a study finding that anethole (main constituent of fennel) inhibited the spread of cancer cells. The study's findings indicated that anethole is a potent anti-metastatic drug. **(D)**

Garlic — The *American Journal of Epidemiology* in January 1994 reported on The Iowa Women's Study, which monitored over 40,000 women, aged 55-69, over 5 years for **colon** cancer incidence. Results from the study showed a strong connection between garlic consumption and **colon** cancer risk. Women who consumed the highest amounts of garlic had a 50% lower risk of cancer of the **distal colon** compared with women who had the lowest level of garlic consumption. **(B)**

In 1998, the *European Journal of Epidemiology* reported on a French case control study involving both pre-menopausal and post-menopausal women between 34-78 years old. The study found increased garlic consumption was associated with a statistically significant reduction in the risk for **breast** cancer. **Breast** cancer risk was notably reduced in those consuming greater amounts of fiber, garlic, and onions. **(B)**

In 2006, the *International Journal of Cancer* reported on a study that was part of the European Prospective Investigation into Cancer and Nutrition (EPIC). EPIC was designed to investigate the relationship among diet, nutritional status, lifestyle and environmental factors and the incidence of cancer and other chronic diseases. It is said to be the largest cohort study on fruit and vegetable intake and the incidence of **stomach** cancer in European countries, having recruited over a half a million people as subjects. Researchers reported that an increase in the intake of onions and garlic of 10 grams per day was associated with a 30% reduction in the risk of **intestinal gastric** cancer. **(B)**

Ginger — In 2007, the journal *Food Chemical Toxicology* published an article noting the 2,500 year history of ginger in medicinal uses across cultures. Additionally, recent research is referenced that indicates that the anti-inflammatory and antioxidant properties of ginger may be useful in preventing cancer. The article noted, "A number of mechanisms that may be involved in the chemopreventive effects of ginger and its components have been reported from the laboratory studies in a wide range of experimental models." **(C)**

Cancer Prevention Research published online in October 2011 the findings of a study funded by the U.S. National Cancer Institute and conducted at the University of Michigan Medical School. It was a very small study involving only 30 people. The preliminary study found that ginger root supplements seem to reduce inflammation in the intestines, which showed that potentially ginger root supplements might reduce the risk of **colon** cancer. The researchers found that the level of inflammation in the subjects who took the ginger pills fell by an average of 28%, as opposed to the subjects that took the placebo. While this was a very small study, the findings were encouraging. **(B)**

Oregano — The Agricultural Research Service reported in the November 2001 issue of the *Journal of Agricultural and Food Chemistry* on a study that tested 27 culinary herbs with an antioxidant test known as ORAC (oxygen radical absorbance capacity). Three types of oregano, Mexican, Italian, and Greek scored highest in antioxidant activity. **(C)**

Rosemary — Critical Reviews in Food Science and Nutrition in December 2011 published an article that reviewed scientific evidence from all studies published from 1996 to March 2010. The studies examined the protective effects of rosemary on **colorectal** and other types of cancer. The studies showed evidence of rosemary to have the ability to suppress the development of tumors in several organs including the **colon**, **breast**, **liver**, and **stomach**, as well as **melanoma** and **leukemia** cells. **(D)**

Thyme — A report in the *British Journal of Nutrition* in 2000 stated that, in a study of rats and thyme oil (more specifically the chemical thymol), rats in the study had higher levels of antioxidants and omega-3 fatty acids as compared to controls. **(D)**

Horseradish — A 2005 study from the University of Illinois shows that glucosinolates, compounds that have been shown to increase human resistance to cancer, are largely present in horseradish. The researchers believe they may even suppress the growth of existing cancerous tumors. **(D)**

In 2009, the *Journal of Agriculture and Food Chemistry* published a study claiming that horseradish has 10 times more glucosinolates than broccoli. As little as less than a teaspoon can be beneficial, according to the scientists. **(D)**

Legumes — Several studies conducted by the American Institute of Cancer Research (AICR) over the last two decades have confirmed that the phytochemicals contained in legumes, including those found in beans, peas, and lentils, have been shown to reduce tumors in laboratory settings. Additionally, these legumes are high in fiber content, which the AICR studies show works to lower the incidence of **colon** cancer. **(D)**

In 2007, the American Institute for Cancer Research and The World Cancer Research Fund's Second Expert Report, Nutrition, Physical Activity, and the Prevention of Cancer: A Global Perspective, found evidence that foods containing dietary fiber, like dry beans and peas (legumes), can lower the risk of certain cancers. They found the strength of the evidence convincing in regards to **colorectal** cancer, and Probable in regards to **pancreatic** cancer. **(C)**

Beans — A 2005 study led by University College, London shows that a chemical compound (inositol pentakisphosphate) found in beans, nuts, and cereals inhibits a key enzyme (phosphoinositide 3-kinase) involved in tumor growth. Additionally, this compound was found to enhance the effect of cytotoxic drugs in **ovarian** and **lung** cancer cells in mice. **(D)**

Black Beans — According to *The Journal of Nutrition*, studies done in 1997 and 2002 showed that rodents fed navy, pinto, and black beans reduced their incidences of **colon** cancer by 52-57%. **(D)**

Nutrition and Cancer in 2002 published the results of a study done at Michigan State University to determine whether consumption of black beans and/or navy beans would reduce **colon** carcinogenesis in rats. It was concluded that eating black beans and navy beans significantly lowered **colon** cancer incidence and multiplicity. **(D)**

Garbanzo Beans (Chickpeas) — The April 1, 2008 edition of the *Journal of Clinical Oncology* published the findings of a Japanese study including 24,226 women ages 40 to 69 who were followed an average of 10 years. The study found those women with the highest intake levels of the isoflavone genistein, plant compounds found in soybeans and garbanzo beans, were only one third as likely to develop **breast** cancer as those without the compound in their systems. Researchers concluded, "Together with past studies, the findings suggest that a high isoflavone intake from food may help lower **breast** cancer risk." **(B)**

Pinto Beans — A recent study by the U.S. Department of Agriculture ranked three varieties of beans in the top four foods studied for antioxidant benefits. Among the three varieties of beans were pinto beans, which ranked higher in antioxidants than many other beans and other fruits and vegetables. **(C)**

A report by nutrition experts at Michigan State University (MSU) reviewed 25 years of bean research and concluded that beans could be a significant asset in helping Americans fight many chronic diseases, including cancer. The report referred to dry-packaged beans in bags and also precooked canned beans, including pinto, navy, kidney, lima and black beans. Their report found, among other facts, that out of 41 countries, those with the highest bean consumption had the lowest death rates from **breast**, **prostate**, and **colon** cancers. **(D)**

Lentils — The April 20, 2005 *International Journal of Cancer* reported that researchers at the Harvard School of Public Health analyzed data from more than 90,000 women who participated in the Nurses' Health Study II. The report showed that people consuming beans or lentils frequently had a 24% lower risk of contracting **breast** cancer than those who did not. **(B)**

Peas — See Legumes above.

Mushrooms — *Cancer Letters* in April 2008 reported on a 2007 study that found clitocine, a natural biologically active substance isolated from the mushroom Leucopaxillus giganteus, possesses several bioactivities including antitumor. Researchers concluded, "Present results suggested that clitotine could be a potential candidate for developing anti-cancer drug for the treatment of human cervical cancer." **(D)**

The journal *Nutrition and Cancer* in 2008 reported on a City of Hope study that found the white button mushroom is particularly effective against **prostate** cancer. Researchers stated, "The data provided by this study illustrate the anticancer potential of phytochemicals in mushroom extract both in vitro and in vivo and supports the recommendation of white button mushroom as a dietary component that may aid in the prevention of **prostate** cancer in men." **(D)**

A report in *Cancer Research*, published online December 18, 2006, reported on research done by researchers at the City of Hope and Ohio State University. Their in vivo studies illustrated that oral intake of mushroom extract suppressed the growth of hormone-dependent **breast** tumors in mice. The researchers concluded, "As this is a pharmacologic dosage that inhibits the growth of established tumor cells in vivo, it is feasible that a lower intake of mushroom ingested regularly as a routine dietary constituent would be effective in preventing the initiation of **breast** tumors in an average woman. **(D)**

Nuts — See Beans above.

Almonds — A study published in 2007 in the *Journal of Agricultural and Food Chemistry* found that the levels of cancer-fighting antioxidants (phenols, flavonoids, and phenolic acids) in a serving of almonds was equal to total polyphenols found in one cup of green tea and one cup of steamed broccoli. **(D)**

Walnuts — The August 2003 issue of *Phytochemistry* reported that researchers had identified 16 polyphenols in walnuts, including three new tannins, with antioxidant activity so powerful they described it as "remarkable." **(D)**

A study published in the journal *Nutrition and Cancer*, September 2008 by a researcher at Marshall University has determined that walnuts are higher in omega-3 fatty acids than any other nuts. In research these fats were shown to reduce existing tumor growth in lab animals and the progression of **breast** cancer tumors by 50%. Walnuts also contain antioxidants and phytosterols that other studies have found to slow cancer. **(D)**

Okra — According to studies conducted at Emory University in Atlanta, Georgia, okra contains glutathione, which acts both as an antioxidant protecting cells from cancer and as a cell "detox" by flushing cancer-causing chemicals from the body. Out of a group of 1,800 people, those who consumed the most glutathione were 50% less likely to develop **oral** and **throat** cancers. **(B)**

A study reported in *Food Chemistry* in 2008 showed through qualitative and quantitative analysis that okra seeds and skins were particularly rich in polyphenolic compounds, mainly composed of quercetin derivatives, and found okra to be an important vegetable for human nutrition. **(D)**

Onions — The *International Journal of Cancer* in July 2006 reported on a case control study conducted in Australia. For females, greater intakes of onions and legumes were associated with decreased risk of **colon** cancer. **(B)**

The *European Journal of Epidemiology* in December 1998 reported on a French study. The study considered total calorie intake and other established risk factors and found that **breast** cancer risk was reduced in those consuming greater amounts of fiber, garlic, and onions. **(B)**

The *American Journal of Clinical Nutrition* in November 2006 reported on results that Italian and Swiss researchers found. In the study they discovered that eating onions appeared to reduce the risk of **colorectal**, **laryngeal**, and **ovarian** cancers. People who ate more onions rather than less also appeared to have less risk of **oral** and esophageal cancers. **(B)**

Peaches — In 2010, the *Journal of Agriculture and Food Chemistry* published reports of a study conducted by AgriLife Research that showed that even aggressive-type **breast** cancer cells were killed after treatment with peach and plum extracts. Normal cells were not killed in the process. The extracts contained phenolic acid components that are found in especially high levels in stone fruits such as peaches and plums. **(D)**

Pears — The World Health Organization and the United States Department of Agriculture research found that cancer risks can be reduced by 20% with a daily intake of at least 5 fruits and vegetables. Research showed that at least 10 fruits can effectively reduce the risk of cancer. Pears were among the top 10 fruits. **(C)**

Pineapple — In a study reported in 2009 in *The Cancer Letter*, scientists at the Indian Institute of Toxicology Research touted the anti-cancer properties of bromelain, the key enzyme in pineapple. Their research with mice reduced **skin** cancer tumors by 65%, and pre-treatment with bromelain reduced the number of tumors occurring at all. **(D)**

Pumpkin — See also Yellow-Orange Vegetables and Fruits.

In 1994, doctors in Tours, France determined that pumpkin fights the metastasis of **breast** cancer. In research reported in the *British Journal of Cancer*, August 1994, they found that women who had levels of alpha-linolenic acid in their tissue were five times less likely to have cancer that spread following surgery than women who had lesser levels. Pumpkin oil is a good source of alpha-linolenic acid. **(B)**

A Harvard University study reported in *The American Journal of Clinical Nutrition* in October 2000 presented findings that pumpkin is a top squash source of beta-cryptoxanthin and alpha-carotene. Subjects with high levels of these chemicals experienced a 63% lower risk of **lung** cancer. **(B)**

Root Vegetables — In 2005, the *International Journal of Cancer* reported on a study performed at the Karolinska Institute in Stockholm that equated regular consumption of root vegetables, including carrots and beets with as high as a 65% decrease in the risk of kidney cancer. **(B)**

Soy — In a study published December 2009 in the *Journal of the American Medical Association* (JAMA), data was analyzed from approximately 5,000 Chinese **breast** cancer survivors, ages 20 to 75. Findings indicated that the higher a woman's intake of soy foods, the lower her chances of cancer (both estrogen-positive and estrogen negative) recurrence and death. **(B)**

Note: According to the American Institute for Cancer Research (AICR), earlier research led to a concern that the isoflavones contained in soy have estrogen-like properties, which might promote the growth of estrogen-based tumors. For this reason, the AICR states, "Current research shows that it is safe to eat moderate amounts of soy foods (e.g., soymilk, tofu), up to 2-3 servings per day. As a precaution, women receiving anti-estrogen treatments such as tamoxifen, should minimize soy foods and avoid isoflavone supplements."

A National Cancer Institute (NCI) study published in *Cancer Epidemiology, Biomarkers and Prevention* reported that women who consumed the highest amounts of soy in childhood had 58% less risk of **breast** cancer compared with those in the lowest groups. When adolescents or adults ate or drank a lot of soy, they found a 20-25% reduction in risk. The relationship between childhood soy consumption and reduced **breast** cancer risk was true for all women in the study, regardless of family history of **breast** cancer. **(B)**

Sprouts — Sulforaphane and diindolylmethane found in broccoli sprouts have been found to inhibit cancer growth, according to Johns Hopkins School of Medicine studies reported in a 1992 report published in the Proceedings of the National Academy of Sciences. **(D)**

Cancer Research reported in 2008 on a study involving broccoli sprout extract administered to rats and found that the extract reduced **bladder** cancer in rats by 70%. The researcher stated: "In conclusion, broccoli sprout extract is a highly promising substance for **bladder** cancer prevention and the isothiocyanates in the extract are selectively delivered to the **bladder** epithelium through urinary excretion." **(D)**

Sweet Potatoes — See also Yellow-Orange Vegetables and Fruits.

In 2004, the *Journal of Agricultural and Food Chemistry* reported on a study by Japanese researchers that determined that extracts of baked sweet potato were high in phenolic compounds, which showed significant scavenging effects against cancer-causing radicals. They also suppressed the proliferation of human myelocytic **leukemia** cells. **(D)**

The journal *Bioscience Biotechnology & Biochemistry* reported in 2005 on research by Indian scientists that found that a significant reduction in **gallbladder** cancer incidence was associated with the consumption of several fruits and vegetables, among them sweet potatoes. This was attributed to the presence of anthocyanins, extract that are strongly antioxidative. **(D)**

Tomatoes — A 2003 Illinois study reported in the *Journal of the National Cancer Institute* found that lycopene, a chemical found in tomatoes, working along with other nutrients in the tomato fruit, led to a reduced incidence of **prostate** cancer in rats. **(D)**

According to the American Cancer Society (www.cancer.org) in a 2012 website notation, "People who have diets rich in tomatoes, which contain lycopene, appear in some studies to have a lower risk of certain types of cancer, especially cancers of the **prostate**, **lung**, and **stomach**. However, not all of the studies have reached the same conclusion. Studies that tested lycopene on men who already had **prostate** cancer have been mixed, but in general found little effect. Further research is needed to find out what role, if any, lycopene has in the prevention or treatment of cancer. It is likely that the preventive effect of diets high in fruits and vegetables cannot be explained by just one single part of the diet." **(C)**

Whole Grains — In December 2005, The Linus Pauling Institute at Oregon State University stated that several case-control studies have shown that diets with a higher whole grain intake help reduce the risk of several types of cancer, including mouth, **throat**, **stomach**, **colon**, and **rectal**. **(C)**

A study published in the *American Journal of Clinical Nutrition* in May of 2007 researched data for almost half a million middle-aged men and women enrolled in the NIH-AARP Diet and Health Study found that diets that include the consumption of whole grains were associated with a modest reduced risk for **colorectal** cancer. The same study also did not find a link between diets that include the consumption of fiber from other food sources and **colorectal** cancer risk. **(B)**

In 2008, the *International Journal of Cancer* published results of a study that suggest that dietary fiber intake from fruit and cereal may play a role in reducing **breast** cancer risk. Over 51,000 postmenopausal women who were studied over an eight-year period showed a 34% reduction in **breast** cancer risk for those consuming the most fruit fiber. Also, in a subgroup of women who had ever used hormone replacement, those consuming the most fiber, especially cereal fiber, showed a 50% reduction in their risk of **breast** cancer. **(B)**

Yellow-Orange Vegetables and Fruits — See also Pumpkins and Sweet Potatoes

A Cornell University study published in *Cancer Research* in July 1998 found that carotenes, the compounds found in a wide assortment of yellow-orange vegetables and fruits, from carrots and sweet potatoes to pumpkins and apricots, caused the body to manufacture retinoic acid, a product of Vitamin A. Retinoic acid reverses mutated genetic material that causes cancer. Cancers such as **leukemia** respond particularly to retinoic acid. Ongoing studies at Cornell University aim to explain exactly how retinoic acid works on oncogenes and whether other, related compounds would be more effective in chemotherapy. Professor Yen, lead researcher, said, "In the meantime I think we're adding evidence that an adequate supply of carotene in the diet is obviously beneficial for anyone who wishes to stay healthy and avoid cancer." **(D)**

Food Study Grading Criteria Glossary

Anecdotal Evidence — The expression anecdotal evidence refers to evidence from a small or "cherry-picked" sample. The term is often used in contrast to those evidences found by the strict application of the scientific method. Some anecdotal evidence does not qualify as scientific evidence because its nature prevents it from being investigated using the scientific method. It is considered evidence, however, although often debatable if accepted, even though it is frequently true and even verifiable. Often it is considered because it is the only evidence we have.

Animal Research — Animal testing, also known as animal experimentation, animal research, and in vivo testing, is the use of non-human animals in experiments. The research is conducted inside universities, medical schools, pharmaceutical companies, farms, defense establishments, and commercial facilities that provide animal-testing services to industry.

Case-control Study — A case-control study is a type of study design used widely, often in epidemiology. Case-control studies are used to identify factors that may contribute to a medical condition by comparing subjects who have that condition/disease (the "cases") with patients who do not have the condition/disease but are otherwise similar (the "controls").

Cohort Study — A cohort study is a research study that compares a particular outcome (such as lung cancer) in groups of individuals who are alike in many ways, but differ by a certain characteristic (for example, female nurses who smoke, compared with those who do not smoke).

Consensus — A consensus is a majority or general agreement of opinion. In science and medicine, this refers to a stated agreement among experts.

Expert — An expert is someone widely recognized as a reliable source of judgment in a given area by their peers or the public.

Epidemiological Study — An epidemiological study is one which examines the distribution and patterns of health-events, health-characteristics, and their causes or influences in well-defined populations. It is designed to identify risk factors for disease and targets for preventive medicine.

Historical Control — A historical control is a control group that is chosen from a group of patients who were observed at some time in the past or for whom data are available through records; HCs are used for comparison with subjects being treated concurrently.

In Vitro — In vitro means in the laboratory (outside the body). It is the opposite of in vivo (in the body).

Meta-analyses — Meta-analyses are processes that analyze data from different studies done about the same subject. The results of a meta-analysis are usually stronger than the results of any study by itself.

Nonrandomized Clinical Trial — A nonrandomized clinical trial is a clinical trial in which the participants are not assigned by chance to different treatment groups. Participants may choose which group they want to be in, or they may be assigned to the groups by the researchers.

Quantitative Data — Quantitative data is any data that is in numerical form such as statistics, percentages, etc. Such data should yield an unbiased result that can be generalized to some larger population.

(RCT) Randomized Clinical Trial — RCTs are also sometimes known as randomized control trials or randomized controlled clinical trials when they concern clinical research. They are studies in which the participants are assigned by chance to separate groups that compare different treatments; neither the researchers nor the participants can choose which group. Using chance to assign people to groups means that the groups will be similar and that the treatments they receive can be compared objectively.

Systematic Review — A systematic review is a review of the literature published on all quality scientific research findings relevant to a particular question. The review utilizes an objective approach to minimize any bias.

Appendix-11

American Cancer Society Guidelines on Nutrition and Physical Activity for Cancer Prevention and Cancer Survivors [1,2]

The American Cancer Society's recommendation for cancer prevention and cancer survivors is to stay away from tobacco, maintain a healthy weight, exercise, limit time spent sitting, and eat fruits, vegetables, and whole grains. They also recommend limiting intake of red meat, processed meats, and alcohol. Please see the American Cancer Society's website for more recommendations. Aside from these basic recommendations, the following are their specific recommendations for specific cancers. Please remember that just because the evidence to support nutrition helping to prevent or fight certain cancers is inconclusive now, that doesn't mean it is definitive. It may or may not mean that this evidence will be produced at a later date with more studies.

Breast Cancer — The best nutrition and physical activity-related advice to reduce the risk of **breast** cancer is to engage in regular, intentional physical activity; to minimize lifetime weight gain through the combination of caloric restriction (in part by consuming a diet rich in vegetables and fruits) and regular physical activity; and to avoid or limit intake of alcoholic beverages.

Colorectal Cancer — The best nutrition and physical activity-related advice to reduce the risk of **colon** cancer is to increase the intensity and duration of physical activity, limit intake of red and processed meat, consume recommended levels of calcium, ensure sufficient Vitamin D status, eat more vegetables and fruits, avoid obesity and central weight gain, and avoid excess alcohol consumption. In addition, it is very important to follow the ACS guidelines for regular colorectal screening, as identifying and removing precursor polyps in the **colon** can prevent **colorectal** cancer.

Endometrial Cancer — At the present time, the best nutrition and physical activity-related advice to reduce the risk of endometrial cancer is to maintain a healthy weight and engage in regular physical activity.

Kidney Cancer — The best nutrition and physical activity-related advice to reduce the risk of kidney cancer is to maintain a healthy weight and avoid tobacco use.

Lung Cancer — The best advice to reduce the risk of lung cancer is to avoid tobacco use and environmental tobacco smoke, and to avoid radon exposure.

Ovarian Cancer — At the present time, the evidence relating nutrition and physical activity to the risk of **ovarian** cancer is inconsistent or limited, although some areas of active research may be promising. No recommendations specific to **ovarian** cancer can be made with confidence.

Pancreatic Cancer — The best advice to reduce the risk of **pancreatic** cancer is to avoid tobacco use and maintain a healthy weight. Physical activity and following the other ACS recommendations related to a healthy diet may also be beneficial.

Prostate Cancer — The best nutrition and physical activity-related advice to reduce the risk of **prostate** cancer is to eat at least 2.5 cups of a wide variety of vegetables and fruits each day, be physically active, and achieve a healthy weight. It may also be prudent to limit calcium supplementation and to not exceed the recommended intake levels of calcium via foods and beverages. However, as calcium and dairy intake may decrease the risk of **colorectal** cancer, the ACS does not make specific recommendations regarding calcium and dairy food intake for overall cancer prevention.

Stomach Cancer — The best advice for reducing the risk of **stomach** cancer is to eat at least 2.5 cups of vegetables and fruits daily; reduce consumption of processed meat, salt, and salt-preserved food; be physically active; and maintain a healthy weight.

Upper Aerodigestive Tract Cancers — These include cancer of the lip, tongue, major salivary glands, gums and adjacent oral cavity tissues, floor of the mouth, tonsils, oropharynx, nasopharynx, hypopharynx, and other oral regions, nasal cavity, accessory sinuses, middle ear, and larynx, cited here: http://www.ncbi.nlm.nih.gov/pubmed/8000993

The best advice to reduce the risk of cancers of the upper digestive and respiratory tracts is to avoid all forms of tobacco, restrict alcohol consumption, avoid obesity, and eat at least 2.5 cups of a variety of vegetables and fruits each day.

1   http://cacancerjournal.com, CA Cancer J Clin 2012;62:30 – 67. VC 2012 American Cancer Society, " American Cancer Society Guidelines on Nutrition and Physical Activity for Cancer Prevention: Reducing the Risk of Cancer With Healthy Food Choices and Physical Activity"

2   acsjournals.com, CA: A Cancer Journal for Clinicians, CA CANCER J CLIN 2012;00:000-000, "Nutrition and Physical Activity Guidelines for Cancer Survivors"

Appendix-III

Summary of the Second Expert Report

Below are the food findings from the Second Expert Report, *Food, Nutrition, Physical Activity, and the Prevention of Cancer: a Global Perspective* published in 2007 by The World Cancer Research Fund (WCRF) and the American Institute for Cancer Research (AICR). It is considered to be the most comprehensive report on diet and cancer completed to date. Also included, drawn from the report, are the 10 recommendations for cancer prevention and percentages of specific cancers that could be avoided with diet, exercise, and weight management.

Initially, over a half million studies were reviewed. They were eventually narrowed down to 7,000 relevant studies, which 21 world-renown scientists then analyzed. It includes information only on foods studied and physical activity. It does not include information regarding supplements or other factors contained within the report. Please note that even though 7,000 studies were analyzed, its conclusions are only as definitive as the available evidence allowed.

Foods That Increase and Decrease Risk for Specific Cancers

Convincing Decreased Risk (strong, consistent, and unlikely to change in the future)
Physical activity (colon)
Foods containing dietary fiber (colon)

Probable Decreased Risk (compelling but not quite strong or consistent enough to be "convincing")
Allium vegetables (stomach)
Foods containing beta-carotene (esophagus)
Foods containing carotenoids (mouth, pharynx, larynx, lung)
Foods containing folate (pancreas)
Foods containing lycopene (prostate)
Foods containing selenium (prostate)
Foods containing Vitamin C (esophagus)
Fruits (mouth, pharynx, larynx, esophagus, lung, stomach)
Garlic (colon)
Milk (colon)
Diets high in calcium (colon)
Non-starchy vegetables (mouth, pharynx, larynx, esophagus, and stomach)
Physical activity (breast postmenopausal, endometrium)
Diets high in calcium (colon)

Limited-Suggestive Decreased Risk (too limited for a grade of "probable," but a general consistency in the data)
Carrots (cervix)
Fish (colon)
Foods containing dietary fiber (esophagus)
Foods containing folate (esophagus, colon)
Foods containing pyridoxine (oesogphagus)
Foods containing quercetin (lung)
Foods containing selenium (lung, stomach, colon)
Food containing Vitamin D (colon)
Foods containing Vitamin E (oesogphagus, prostate)
Fruits (nasopharynx, pancreas, liver, colon)
Milk (bladder)
Non-starchy vegetables (nasopharynx, lung, colon, ovary, and endometrium)
Pulses (legumes) (stomach, prostate)
Physical activity (lung, pancreas, breast premenopausal)

Convincing Increased Risk (strong, consistent, and unlikely to change in the future)
Red meat (colon)
Processed meat (colon)
Arsenic in drinking water (lung)
Alcoholic drinks (mouth, pharynx, larynx, esophagus, (colon, men), breast premenopause, breast postmenopause)

Probable Increased Risk (compelling but not quite strong or consistent enough to be "convincing")
Cantonese-style salted fish (nasopharynx)
Diets high in calcium (prostate)
Fast foods (weight gain, overweight, and obesity)
Maté (esophagus)
Alcoholic drinks (liver) (colon, women)
Salt (stomach)
Salted and salty foods (stomach)

Limited-Suggestive Increased Risk (too limited for a grade of "probable," but a general consistency in the data)
Chili (stomach)
Red meat (esophagus, lung, pancreas, endometrium)
Processed meat (esophagus, lung, stomach, prostate)
Foods containing iron (colon)
Smoked foods (stomach)
Grilled or barbequed animal foods (stomach)
Milk and dairy products (prostate)
Cheese (colon)
Total Fat (lung, breast postmenopause)
Foods containing animal fat (colon)
Butter (lung)
Foods containing sugars (colon)
Maté (mouth pharynx, larynx)
High temperature drinks (esophagus)

Substantial Effect on Risk Unlikely (enough evidence to rule out a connection)
Foods containing beta-carotene (prostate, skin)
Coffee (pancreas, kidney)
Alcoholic drinks (kidney)

    In addition, the expert panel recommends staying away from foods and drinks that promote weight gain, i.e., sugary drinks, fast foods, and energy-dense foods. (Energy density measures the amount of energy per weight in food. Processed foods that contain considerable amounts of fat or sugar tend to be more energy-dense than fresh foods.)

Ten Recommendations for Cancer Prevention (as listed on the AICR website)
1. Be as lean as possible without becoming underweight.
2. Be physically active for at least 30 minutes every day.
3. Avoid sugary drinks. Limit consumption of energy-dense foods.
4. Eat more of a variety of vegetables, fruits, whole grains and legumes such as beans.
5. Limit consumption of red meats (such as beef, pork, and lamb) and avoid processed meats.
6. If consumed at all, limit alcoholic drinks to 2 for men and 1 for women a day.
7. Limit consumption of salty foods and foods processed with salt (sodium).
8. Don't use supplements to protect against cancer.
9. *It is best for mothers to breastfeed exclusively for up to 6 months and then add other liquids and foods.
10. *After treatment, cancer survivors should follow the recommendations for cancer prevention.
*Special Population Recommend

Index